T0176312

"Beautifully written and passionately reported, *The Long Haul* is an essential insight into how Covid-19's effects could be with us for decades. Expertly chronicling the lives of these survivors, Ryan Prior shows us the dedication of hero physicians and the strength of empowered patients who stick up for themselves to get the best care. Most important, it gives us a front-row seat for how groups of long haulers are harnessing their power to organize for a health care system that works better for all of us."
—ELIZABETH COHEN, Senior Medical Correspondent, CNN; author of *The Empowered Patient*

"Ryan Prior's years of both living with and reporting on chronic disease for major publications makes him ideally suited to write a book about Long Covid. Because he has led the field by helping author principles guiding other science writers in covering contested diseases, he can cover this topic with all the scientific nuance, literary poise, and human empathy it requires. His book could be an example in future decades of how to cover the new epidemics we will undoubtedly see."
—PAM WEINTRAUB, former Executive Editor, *Discover*; author of *Cure Unknown: Inside the Lyme Epidemic*

"Everyone needs to read this book. Every one of us will either experience Long Covid or have a loved one who experiences it. *The Long Haul* is a story that needs to be told right now by the person who needs to tell it. It's a deeply moving and beautifully written account of the quest by patients to unlock the unknowns of Long Covid and provide a roadmap for overcoming many of the twenty-first century's problems."
—DR. DAVID FAJGENBAUM, Immunologist, University of Pennsylvania; national bestselling author of *Chasing My Cure: A Doctor's Race to Turn Hope Into Action*

"In reading *The Long Haul* by Ryan Prior, I learned a lot about Covid long haulers. Ryan covered the history and the remarkable patients that brought this disease to the public, government, and medical awareness. I agree with Ryan that researchers need to be very aware of the research done on other postviral illnesses, especially ME/CFS. It's a remarkable story and Ryan is an interesting and creative writer."
—RON DAVIS, Professor of Biochemistry and Genetics, Stanford University; inventor of technologies fueling the Human Genome Project

"Journalist Ryan Prior's major account of Long Covid, *The Long Haul*, is superb. Along with meditative sidebars on science and medicine, Prior offers a wide-ranging investigation into the history, science, and politics of this chronic condition—potentially the fate of one in five Covid survivors. Prior's street cred as both a Long Covid survivor and a victim of myalgic encephalomyelitis (ME), a decades-old chronic disease to which some compare Long Covid, renders him a compassionate, insightful narrator."
—HILLARY JOHNSON, author of *Osler's Web: Inside the Labyrinth of the Chronic Fatigue Syndrome Epidemic*

"Ryan Prior's passion to both get the story right and bring it alive using amazing storytelling skills makes his work incredibly important and engaging. His experience living with chronic illness and his years of writing about it will all combine to make his book on Long Covid an essential read."
—TRACIE WHITE, author of *The Puzzle Solver: A Scientist's Quest to Cure the Illness that Stole His Son*

THE LONG

HAUL

How Long Covid Survivors Are
Revolutionizing Healthcare

RYAN PRIOR

The MIT Press
Cambridge, Massachusetts
London, England

For Mom, Dad, Pam Stanescu, and Cindy Shepler

The MIT Press would like to thank the anonymous peer reviewers who provided comments on drafts of this book. The generous work of academic experts is essential for establishing the authority and quality of our publications. We acknowledge with gratitude the contributions of these otherwise uncredited readers.

This book was set in Minion Pro. Printed and bound in the United States of America.

Library of Congress Cataloging-in-Publication Data

Names: Prior, Ryan, author.
Title: The long haul : how long covid survivors are revolutionizing
   healthcare / Ryan Prior.
Description: Cambridge, Massachusetts : The MIT Press, [2024] | Includes
   bibliographical references.
Identifiers: LCCN 2023030212 | ISBN 9780262548151 (paperback)
Subjects: MESH: Post-Acute COVID-19 Syndrome | Chronic Disease—therapy |
   Delivery of Health Care—trends | Patient Participation | Personal
   Narrative
Classification: LCC RA644.C67 | NLM WC 506.5 | DDC
   362.1962/4144—dc23/eng/20230908
LC record available at https://lccn.loc.gov/2023030212

10   9   8   7   6   5   4   3   2   1

"Disease is very old, and nothing about it has changed. It is we who change, as we learn to recognize what was formerly imperceptible."

JEAN-MARTIN CHARCOT, *De l'expectation en médecine*

Contents

PREFACE TO THE
PAPERBACK EDITION

IN PERHAPS JOHN F. KENNEDY'S most enduring speech, our thirty-fifth president lays down one of history's great challenges: "We choose to go to the Moon in this decade and do the other things not because they are easy but because they are hard."

In the decades since, the term "moonshot" has become shorthand for taking on the most daunting, yet worthy, scientific endeavors. In medicine, researchers have announced moonshots to tackle cancer and arthritis. These are impossible, *wicked* problems.

Beyond the dramatic human tragedy they seek to resolve, moonshot thinking has a larger purpose for how we think about science and society. In Kennedy's speech, he argues that landing on the moon matters "because that goal will serve to organize and measure the best of our energies and skills."

During the Covid-19 pandemic, our most important "moonshot" was Operation Warp Speed, a public–private partnership that accomplished the fastest vaccine rollout in history. It organized the best of our energies and skills.

These impossible projects can succeed when thousands of people are aligned on a mission, when we pursue it with diligence and generosity of spirit, and when society offers up the resources and incentives to achieve explosive innovation. So throughout writing *The Long Haul*, these ideas were constantly in my mind. Long Covid and its cousins are thorny, knotty problems. To solve the problem at scale, they require a battlefield general, a mass organizer. They may well require a brand new paradigm for thinking about medicine. They certainly require a moonshot.

In the months after this book was released, I took a full-time job at a think tank, joined a telehealth startup as an advisor, and got to work on a syllabus to teach a course on science writing at Georgia State University. I launched a column called "Patient Revolution" with *Psychology Today*. I was invited to speak to federal agencies about how to innovate in the healthcare system. I served on committees looking into finding a biomarker for complex diseases. I kept up a constant stream of articles, including a feature in *The Nation* entitled "The Long Covid Revolution," written alongside Fiona Lowenstein, a visionary writer and Long Covid activist you'll meet in chapter three.

Fiona and I laid out a list of public policies that can address Long Covid. Some of those ideas include establishing a fund to pay for long haulers' medical costs, like the September 11 Victim Compensation Fund. We argued for public funding to community-level organizations that can disseminate crucial information about prevention, care, and access to testing or treatment. That's vital to build out a resilient healthcare infrastructure that can manage the inevitable long-haul consequences of any future pandemic as well. Fiona and I also called for the National Institutes of Health to create a new office dedicated to studying infection-associated chronic illnesses. If there were to be a true moonshot to solve complex, chronic diseases, I believe this office could very well be the launchpad. The government alone can provide the upfront investment, along with the incumbent resources, coordination, and long-term vision.

But even more important than that, I believe, the Long Covid movement shows the moral imagination for how this seemingly "new" disease fits into the larger American tradition of campaigning for civil rights, women's rights, and LGBT rights. We believe that Covid long haulers are reinvigorating the next generation of the disability rights movement.

I now work every day as a journalist-in-residence at the Century Foundation, alongside Rebecca Vallas, whom you'll meet in chapter 14. In that same chapter, you'll read words from a Rose Garden speech by President Joe Biden announcing that Covid long haulers are entitled to protections under the Americans with Disabilities Act. That raft of policies was coordinated by his director of disability policy, Kim Knackstedt, whom Rebecca also recruited to join the Century Foundation. We all now work together in organizing the Disability Economic Justice Collaborative, a coalition of more than forty think tanks and grassroots organizations charting the future of disability policy.

I have been heartened by the Biden administration's national research action plan for Long Covid and his administration's early efforts to stand up an Office of Long Covid in the Department of Health and Human Services. But along with much of the patient community, I've been critical of bureaucracies that can't move at the urgency needed by patients—especially those at the margins of society—who don't have access to a single FDA-approved drug and who are falling through the cracks in a system that was woefully unprepared even before the pandemic.

My original hope, a cure, still remains a dream. More than 100 million patients around the world may still be suffering, navigating a medical system that does not have good answers for them. It breaks my heart that I can't offer any immediate solace. But I take refuge in the notion that this moment represents a generational pivot point. And over the next one, three, and ten years, the steady work of thousands of scientists, journalists, activists, policymakers, and entrepreneurs will bend the arc of history.

Even more than finding a cure for chronic illnesses, my ultimate mission for this book was always to tell the story of how a group of people with a problem can organize, step up, and chart a necessary solution. I believe this book documents that struggle of the fighters "in the arena," as Teddy Roosevelt would say, "whose face is marred by dust and sweat and blood; who strives valiantly." That attitude is integral to progress, knowing that if we fail, it only comes "while daring greatly."

As you read, I encourage you to let this book challenge you and inspire you to think about how science and society can solve any complex problem. And I hope you will dedicate your life to tackling an impossible challenge.

Chapter 1

A FUTURE
IN JEOPARDY

IT ISN'T JUST LIFE OR death. Even a mild case of the virus can disable many of us for the rest of our lives. And our leaders had no idea.

That thought hung in the back of my mind on the last day of February 2020, while I was working a weekend shift filling in as a breaking news writer for CNN's Ticker, drafting updates on global events that scrolled across the bottom of millions of viewers' screens. From the video feed at my desk in the main newsroom of CNN's world headquarters in Atlanta, I watched as Vice President Mike Pence stepped to the podium in the White House briefing room to give an update on that morning's two-and-a-half-hour meeting of the White House Coronavirus Task Force. After his opening statement, Pence introduced Alex Azar, the Secretary of Health and Human Services, who sought to assure the public that the administration had the outbreak under control and that the risk to the average American from the virus was low.

"It's important to remember," Azar said, "for the vast majority of individuals who contract the novel coronavirus, they will experience mild to moderate symptoms, and their treatment will be to remain at home, treating their symptoms the way they would a severe cold or the flu."

He continued: "For some individuals, a smaller percentage, especially those who may be medically fragile, they will require medical attention including, possibly, hospitalization."

His stable demeanor and cool command of the room belied more stubborn truths brewing behind what we now know was an emergent global pandemic. For my own part, I dwelled on something much different from what most people were concerned with as I took in Azar's words: I was thirty years old at the time. At first glance, I might have looked like one of the strong young people we imagined with immune cells that could easily stare down the crown-shaped virus circulating the globe. But like seven million others in the U.S., I was immunocompromised.

I knew that if I were infected with the coronavirus, it could mean much more than two weeks of illness at home. Although it might not kill me, it might threaten every ambition I held for my professional career and every dream of one day being a husband and a father.

Over the following month, I would aid in CNN's coverage of the pandemic from various vantage points. In my role as a Cross-Platform Associate Producer, I trained across half a dozen different teams, including the Ticker, Special Projects, and a variety of roles as a digital writer in the newsroom. Flexibility right down to the moment was often the number one priority of the role. Based on the network's needs, I could be called to contribute in any number of ways.

On March 11, 2020, due to a gap in my schedule, I had a training day shadowing a producer on the *Anderson Cooper 360°*

show team. During the eight-hour shift, the producer frequently used sanitizing wipes to clean every inch of the workstation in the small edit bay where we sat. Much of the day was spent preparing for President Donald Trump's address to the nation from the Oval Office. There was speculation that he would call a national emergency that evening to empower the nation to deal with the unprecedented threat.

We sat in silence, just after 9 p.m., as Trump explained his administration's new policy: "To keep new cases from entering our shores, we will be suspending all travel from Europe to the United States for the next thirty days." Much of the speech was tied up in an attempt to project a Reaganesque optimism, broadcasting the idea the virus was no match for the greatest nation on earth.

"If we are vigilant—and we can reduce the chance of infection, which we will—we will significantly impede the transmission of the virus," Trump said. "The virus will not have a chance against us. No nation is more prepared or more resilient than the United States. We have the best economy, the most advanced health-care, and the most talented doctors, scientists, and researchers anywhere in the world." Commentators opined that the policy was wrong, that the tone was off, that we were not mobilizing fast enough.

That night as I walked out of the CNN Center, a building to which I'd reported nearly every day for five years, I didn't realize that as the whole company shifted to working from home, it would be seventeen months before I set foot in the office again.

A week later, I began what would become a year-long assignment as a features writer for CNN primarily focused on science, health, and wellness. My first day in that role was also the whole network's first day of remote work. As with nearly everyone on earth, just about every conversation I would have over the next year revolved around the virus. Every country and institution, large and small, would spend that year negotiating their roles and lobbying for resources. Every news site would overflow with analyses on these topics, and countless books would be written about each aspect of the response, or lack thereof. I couldn't and can't espouse expertise on all of minutiae of immunology and epidemiology, but there is one area where I do consider myself an expert: I have lived with a long-term illness following an infection for more than fifteen years. And since the start of the pandemic, I have told the stories of those with similar experiences due to Covid-19. While most of the nation's attention was paid to case counts and death counts and the swirling controversies around lockdowns, school closures, and mask mandates, I felt compelled to bear witness on behalf of millions who felt voiceless after not only becoming infected with the virus, but suffering disabling symptoms for months, and sometimes years, afterwards.

On the night of his Oval Office address, Trump focused his comments toward "the vast majority of Americans," explaining that "the risk is very, very low. Young and healthy people can expect to recover fully and quickly if they should get the virus." I knew those words to be inadequate then. And over the ensuing months, I would continually publish stories reporting on a growing group of survivors who would come to be called Covid-19 "long haulers."

It would turn out to be true that the majority of patients infected with the virus would get better quickly, but that number would fall short of being the *vast* majority. Public health leaders' early comments about most people getting better, which reflected the prevailing public belief at the time, didn't begin to capture the full picture of the disaster that would happen in the lives of many of the pandemic's survivors.

In the weeks after lockdowns began, I received a disquieting message from Linda Tannenbaum, executive director of the Open Medicine Foundation, a non-profit organization in California dedicated to funding research for complex chronic diseases. She'd been a friend and a source for my stories for nearly a decade. The scientists her organization worked with were prestigious forward thinkers, and she was alarmed at what they could already see. She confided that she expected the novel coronavirus, which had been designated SARS-CoV-2, could cause years or even decades of disability in some sufferers. So many other long-time sources reached out with the same warning that I began to dread picking up my phone.

Covid-19 had its predecessor in the first severe acute respiratory syndrome (SARS) virus, which mainly terrorized Asia in the early years of the new millennium. For many patients, Tannenbaum explained, that virus had left years of wreckage in its wake. A 2009 study of 369 SARS survivors published in *JAMA Internal Medicine* showed that four years after initial infection, some 40 percent had a chronic fatigue problem, and 27 percent met the Centers for Disease Control and Prevention's diagnostic criteria for chronic fatigue syndrome. If the second SARS virus—which causes Covid-19—were to prove as wicked in the long term as the first, it might mean years of disability for a swath of humanity. Knowing chronic illness so intimately already, I could barely let myself process or imagine the scope of the pain. Having met hundreds of post-viral patients prior to the Covid-19 pandemic, I considered the prospect of a mass disabling event very likely.

And looking at scientific literature about previous epidemics, I saw similar trends in history. Before researcher Jonas Salk pioneered a vaccine in the 1950s that led to the disease being virtually eradicated, the polio virus fueled terrifying outbreaks around the world for millennia, accounting for many deaths among children and causing irreversible paralysis in about 1 in 200 patients. But, less commonly acknowledged, the virus also caused post-polio syndrome in 25 to 40 percent of survivors, leading to muscle aches and fatigue that could last for decades. Likewise, the Ebola virus, which caused more than twenty-eight thousand cases during its 2014–2016 epidemic, left its own post-viral syndrome. During that outbreak, Ebola killed more than a third of those it infected, and more than 70 percent of survivors were left with a constellation of symptoms including headaches, joint pain, fatigue, and menstrual cessation.

In 2020, as healthcare systems around the world were overwhelmed with dying patients, thousands of very sick people dealing with the ongoing effects of Covid-19 began gathering in online support groups offering each other guidance as months passed and their expected recovery never came.

In July, the CDC released a study of 292 Covid-19 patients showing that 35 percent of them still had symptoms after two or three weeks; among younger people between ages 18 and 34, about one in five included in the study had not fully recovered. Assuming that data generalized to the wider population, it was evidence showing that Covid-19 could linger beyond its two-week recovery time and long-term symptoms were a possibility.

The next month, a science writer colleague sent me a study from the United Kingdom that burned itself into my consciousness. It appeared to show that about three-quarters of those hospitalized for Covid-19 experienced symptoms beyond the twelve-week mark. Another long hauler symptom study out of the UK, which has now tracked five million patients via a symptom tracking app, showed that one in ten people were sick for at least three weeks.

The fears that my sources and friends had expressed to me were being realized.

But hope—seemingly irrational at the time—hung at the edge of each of these conversations.

It was becoming clear that studying why some people get sick, and stay sick, could be one of the greatest scientific opportunities of our lifetime.

DISEASE IS VERY OLD AND NOTHING ABOUT IT HAS CHANGED

A week before my seventeenth birthday, on October 22, 2006, I came home from school and slept for sixteen hours. I did this again and again, day after day. We didn't know what was wrong, and it wasn't getting better. After two weeks I had to quit going to school altogether. The rest of my junior year was consumed with home visits from teachers to carry me through my AP classes and doctor's appointments through which my family and I desperately sought not just a cure for my illness, but simply a diagnosis. After visits to sixteen doctors, what felt like every possible medical test, and failed hypotheses including HIV, mononucleosis, and bipolar disorder, we were still at a loss.

The symptoms were wide and varied. Over the weeks and months, my body almost always felt heavy. I had constant headaches and muscle aches. The smallest stimulation in sound or light would overwhelm me. The most minimal stressor could throw me into a "crash" for hours. Lying in bed, there were often times when even lifting my head up for a few minutes sapped all of my strength. Resting in absolute stillness in a dark room, I structured my life to preserve every last sliver of energy in order to accomplish only the most important tasks, letting every other worry or plan or goal fall away. Many automatic functions of my body never seemed reliable. I would feel ravenous, but when I tried to eat the food disgusted me. My body felt like it had ceased to be able to create energy, and yet some days I couldn't sleep at all. When I could sleep, I didn't feel refreshed at all. Predicting day by day, or hour by hour, whether I'd be functional was impossible.

Basic thinking and comprehension were often fleeting. In one unmooring memory, I recall looking at a stop sign while driving, aware there were letters on it, but not knowing the concept they expressed.

In my small town of Warner Robins, Georgia, my friends in high school joked that when I was finally diagnosed, doctors would call the illness "Ryan Prior disease." But after six months, the label was simply "chronic fatigue syndrome," a diagnosis of exclusion or a so-called "wastebasket diagnosis" used when symptoms can't be attributed to a known disease. I was told the term just implied the absence of any identifiable cause for a condition that had totally derailed my life.

I pushed, and sometimes hobbled, my way through the University of Georgia taking twenty pills a day, giving myself a shot weekly, and driving four hours round trip each month to receive an infusion, all of which wasn't covered by medical insurance. As a college senior studying English and international affairs, I wrote a story for *USA Today* about the illness that changed my life. It garnered a flood of messages from around the world. I learned that the history of my strange disease was far more complicated than I realized, and that I was far from unique. After graduation, I raised $150,000, created a non-profit organization, and built a film production team. We set off on a journey around the country, from Harvard to Stanford to Columbia, directing a documentary film about what I would come to feel was a forgotten plague.

What we had originally thought of as "Ryan Prior disease," and later as chronic fatigue syndrome, was actually myalgic encephalomyelitis, or ME/CFS, a complex neuro-immune disease affecting between 836,000 and 2.5 million Americans and between 17-24 million people worldwide. However, the Food and Drug Administration had not approved a specific drug to treat the underlying condition and still hasn't today. And ME/CFS was receiving just $5 million annually in National Institutes of Health research funding. Despite major constraints, however, researchers had published thousands of peer-reviewed papers about ME/CFS, which they characterized as being as *severe* as late-stage AIDS, multiple sclerosis, and kidney failure.

The disease often appears following a moderate or severe viral or bacterial infection, likely set off by a genetic or other predisposition that scientists are still teasing out. Years after I fell ill, tests revealed that my own case might have been triggered by a Lyme disease infection, likely from a tick bite at a Boy Scout camp when I was sixteen.

I became familiar with the chore of giving countless vials of my own blood. As a writer thrust into science journalism by my own personal health crisis, I also became well-versed with interviewing top experts and steeping myself in medical literature and the political controversies around how diseases are framed, named, and funded. It was a skill and perspective I never wanted, but it became useful in telling stories the world needs to hear.

Our documentary film, medical advocacy, and my ambitions as a journalist led me to becoming a writer for CNN in my mid-twenties, frequently focusing on how patients had transformed their own lives, and those of others, by innovating new treatments when they hit a wall in the medical system.

I wrote about Stanford's Ron Davis, who pioneered the technology that fueled the Human Genome Project, but then transformed his research career in his seventies to pursue a cure for his son, who lost the ability to talk or eat solid food due to myalgic encephalomyelitis. I profiled Doug Lindsay, a college dropout who was bedridden for eleven years with a rare autonomic condition before inventing a new surgery and curing himself. And I put together a series of features on Dr. David Fajgenbaum, a medical student with Castleman disease, which presents with characteristics akin to cancer and autoimmune disease. He nearly died five times from the severe cytokine storms it caused. At one point his family brought a priest into his hospital room to perform last rites. Yet he learned he could repurpose a drug for his disease, saved his own life, and now runs a clinical trial bringing that drug to others with Castleman.

Telling their stories was a way of also telling a version of my own: it helped me understand the depths of what had happened to me and how to channel that experience into helping as many people as possible.

With each story I wrote, I felt I was tapping into a set of principles about how regular people faced with horrific or unforgiving circumstances can transform their own lives. Even more impressive, these same people who lost faith in mainstream medical dogma miraculously had enough faith in themselves to keep fighting. They pursued their own intuition, many times despite doubt and abandonment from family, friends, and medical providers. I had a voracious craving to tell these stories in the hope that they might augur new ways of being in our own bodies and believing in our own capacity to seek insights, build teams, and guide change both within the medical system and in the wider world.

Then a global pandemic hit.

As Covid-19 spread around the world, my inbox lit up with e-mails from sources I've interviewed and collaborated with over the last six or seven years. Each source had a message that scared me, that stole my sleep, and that told me I may need to conjure up all my talent to embrace a new mission in my life. Covid-19 would be a global viral pandemic, but it would likely spark its own second chronic disease pandemic for post-viral sufferers whose lives could be upended for decades. And we would need knowledgeable storytellers to delve into the scientific nuance with grace and empathy, so that Covid-19 long haulers didn't face the same decades of controversy that had mired progress in diseases like my own.

Most importantly, if patients, scientists, policymakers, and journalists each rose to the challenge, we might finally solve the most intractable immune-related diseases that have gnawed at the edges of our health system. This is a vital chance to be bold. We are now in the midst of a polio-like epidemic of long-term disability. Within the first two years of the pandemic, scientists projected there were up to 100 million long haulers worldwide. Many of them experience cognitive illness that resembles brain injury, which leaves the possibility of a later epidemic of neurodegenerative diseases such as dementia and Parkinson's years down the road.

Working together, it's possible to define, treat, and defeat Long Covid. And in the process, we might be able to end the years of misunderstanding endured by those with diseases such as chronic Lyme, ME/CFS, Gulf War syndrome, fibromyalgia, multiple chemical sensitivities, or postural orthostatic tachycardia syndrome. As with Long Covid, the underlying pathology of each of these diseases is hard to detect, the scientific base isn't well developed, and patients are often told their symptoms are all in their head. Covid-19 is a once-in-a-century pandemic, but it's also a once-in-a-century opportunity to leverage public awareness and political capital into finally building a true understanding of post-viral and autoimmune illness.

This book is the true story of people fighting a disease.

Their lives resonate achingly closely with my own. Covid-19 long haulers are like canaries in a coal mine, people whose experiences we can peel back to reveal important insights about our immune systems, our medical system, and our common humanity.

Illness and disease are universal in the human experience. It's not a question of if, but rather *when*, frailty might strike us. And often it's at a younger age than we would have envisioned. More than 150 million Americans, or about 40 percent of us, have a chronic disease. I've claimed my own form of citizenship in that tribe for more than a decade. Millions of Americans will join this group as a result of their Covid complications. One of the most important questions long haulers can ask the world is whether Covid-19 complications are random or whether they strike particularly acutely in patients with particular environmental, genetic, or epigenetic profiles.

In many people, the illness is already irrevocably altering their lives by dimming their ambitions, decimating their finances, and shattering their relationships. It exerts a weight across families and communities, with caregivers often bearing the brunt, physically or psychically, in ways that can almost come to rival the pain of the actual sufferer.

Illness dramatically redirected my own life too. I still suffer relapses, on a roughly annual basis that can leave me bedbound for weeks.

I rely on the help of a rare specialist and a robust treatment plan that requires swallowing dozens of pills per day. But after a couple years in college, I had recovered to the point of being in a form of remission more often than not. In the intervening decade, I found that disease exists in the space between the person we are and the person we'd like to be. Part of *reclaiming* selfhood meant picking items off my bucket list, dreams I'd held long before I became sick, and which straddled the schism in my psyche between pre- and post-illness selves. As an adult I spent hours thinking of the person I had wanted to be when I was in junior high, and many of those visions were simply experiences to be had. In frequent periods when my health felt unstable, the idea of travel often felt too risky: a bit of jet lag or a chaotic sleeping arrangement overseas could carry with it the specter of relapse, threatening my ability to make it through school or hold down a job. But as the illness subsided into near remission, the existential fear of jagged downturns held less sway over my future decisions. There was little standing in my way path toward seeking adventure.

So, as I settled into my career, I eventually gained the confidence to set off on a road trip with a friend down the Pacific Coast Highway, ticking off one of those long-held dreams. I kept going. I'll never forget the moment when I first saw the Eiffel Tower sparkling at night. Also emblazoned in memory is the moment when I was in Rome chatting with a taxi driver, and I fell quiet as I shifted to the other side of the car to take in the Colosseum, which was even more awe-inspiring than I had imagined. Those were moments of wonder. They were also moments of healing, of uniting past and present versions of myself.

Whatever our dreams, they are the fuel that can power us through sustained illness, and they are far more important than the incremental ups and downs of lab tests and medication changes. It may be impossible to truly get back to who we were before getting sick. Repairing that breach, for me, meant relentlessly pursuing the right specialist, holding healthcare providers accountable, garnering support from family and friends, and doggedly adhering to a medical regimen. It also requires a total reassessment of one's expectations for life, combined with a daring faith to hold true to the goals that are still possible.

"First, do no harm" is perhaps the most widely known principle in medical ethics. But there's another concept that I believe is nearly as sacred, which risks being lost in a world of over-reliance on diagnostic testing—particularly those tests that are unreliable for Long Covid and similar complex diseases in which science is contested or emerging—and our often too bureaucratic healthcare system. It comes from the nineteenth-century scholar Sir William Osler, beloved by medical students as a dean of medical education. *Believe patients*, he preached to new trainee doctors. "Listen to your patient. He is telling you the diagnosis." By entering into the world of long haulers, we're challenged to absorb the full gravity of their suffering and to use that wisdom to not only to reframe our view of the pandemic or of healthcare, but also to spark change in all of us. The virus, in its many variants, has inextricably shifted our collective future. The world we rebuild must empower the potentially continuous pipeline of wounded survivors to retain their dignity.

The goal of "medicine" is to cure disease, yes, but even more than that, it is to embrace the sick and to give them back the sacred gift of being able to dream.

This is a story about getting the medical system to work for you in the face of a disease that defies categorization. Multisystem diseases are anti-bureaucratic. Bureaucracies choke on them. It's also a story of the dignity of the sick. In a world in which doctors can often be too overwhelmed to be able to follow the latest trends in specialized research, patients can rise to be the experts in their own diseases. And those who've endured deep suffering can impart profound wisdom to the world, shaping policies for people whom they've never met and even those who have yet to be born.

Chapter 2

A SURPRISING
PROBLEM

"What does it feel like?"

As our cities went into lockdown, the question pulled at our collective curiosity: if we fell ill, would it be just a passing cold, or would the virus take us to the threshold of death? Might it change us forever?

In my reporting, I began piecing together a montage of how Covid-19's long tail affected people around the world, from babies as young as two years old to those in their seventies, regardless of race, class, or background. Lingering effects were particularly glaring in those who had never experienced chronic illness. It was startling how widespread the long tail illness was, how it simmered just beneath the surface, not fully accounted for in the constant news of coronavirus deaths and case counts. So many people were caught off guard by what they thought would be only a couple weeks of severe illness.

In those first few months of the pandemic, I started writing feature stories about the human impact of the virus, getting in touch with dozens of people with long-term symptoms struggling to return to previously vibrant lives. I spoke to a television writer whose credits include *Saturday Night Live* and *The Tonight Show Starring Jimmy Fallon*. "I have to use an inhaler every couple of minutes to reinvigorate my lungs," she told me.

Even short conversations were a struggle for her. "I hear it in my voice just talking to you," she said in a phone interview. "I'm winded."

I met a thirteen-year-old girl in Massachusetts who played on multiple basketball teams at the same time and dreamed of playing in the WNBA, but who even six months after the infection could barely walk for ten minutes.

There was a hair stylist in Aurora, Colorado with three children who all got sick. Her baby's veins were visible through her skin. "It's in her circulatory system. It's like my kids are see-through," she said.

In September of 2020, I spoke to two teenage sisters in Idaho who made several trips to the emergency room, but who had trouble being taken seriously because they couldn't get Covid tests early on in the pandemic.

"Doctors will say one thing to your face, but they won't treat you by what they say," one of the sisters, a high school senior, told me. "It's like they're lying and saying, 'Yes, you have Covid, but no, I won't do anything about it.' It makes you feel powerless."

Due to severe testing shortages across the nation early in the pandemic, many people who experienced acute Covid-19 symptoms—along with their long-term aftermath—do not have a definitive test showing they actually ever had a coronavirus infection in the first place. Lacking a singular data point to start from makes it more difficult for them to get doctors to believe them, and more difficult to gain traction in the quest for reimbursement for care from their insurance companies.

While there is no demographic exempt from the physical, emotional, and economic impact of the Covid-19 pandemic, we do know that the pandemic widened already existing health disparity gaps for many vulnerable populations. A growing body of research shows that people below the federal poverty level, those in prison, people in essential jobs or who could not work from home, people of color, uninsured people, those with pre-existing conditions, undocumented migrants, the elderly, and LGBTQ people were disproportionately affected by Covid-19 and the social and economic effects of the pandemic.

As people within these groups inevitably contract Long Covid, experts worry they will be further alienated as they face additional economic and social barriers, resulting in even less access to care. Given a particular population's underlying health, more severe outcomes occurred in communities of color, according to the CDC. American Indian and Alaska natives who contracted Covid were more than three times more likely to be hospitalized due to the virus than the general American population, and Latino and Black populations were more than twice as likely to end up in the hospital. Even gathering accurate and equitable data about the problem is a project that tests every blind spot of our healthcare system.

One of our great responsibilities as a society is to recognize the ways in which the virus has indelibly etched itself into these millions of bodies, transfiguring them into living fossils of a contagion that changed the world forever.

A ROLL CALL OF LIVES ON HOLD

Behind every statistic is a face. Behind every data point is a life torn asunder not just by the long-term illness, but by fear and uncertainty.

Amy Carrillo, a forty-three-year-old from Kansas, was sobbing alone in March 2020 two weeks into her Covid infection. Her eight-year-old daughter walked in, asking if she was going to die. All Carrillo could do was hold her girl and cry and tell her she hoped the answer was no. The virus didn't take Amy Carrillo's life, but throughout the next year it took much of who she was.

Carrillo had been an avid reader and was always working her way through two or three books at a time, a vital respite she used to stay centered and grounded while working in sales and raising her kids. But Covid stole her ability to concentrate. She couldn't read for nearly a year after contracting the virus. Before Covid, Carrillo had completed a Half Ironman triathlon—a 1.2-mile swim, 56-mile bike ride, and 13.1-mile run—*all while pregnant with her fourth child*. The disease humbled her, however, turning just walking around the block into a struggle. She managed to run a handful of times over the next year and a half, but each time it sent her into a relapse.

"It was, and is, lonely, frightening, and maddening," she told me. "And then we have to deal with BS from anti-vaxxers, anti-maskers, and Covid deniers on top of losing our health and identity."

Carrillo had to focus on learning to summon uncommon levels of patience and forgiveness toward herself as she continued on a path toward hopeful healing that often wasn't linear.

"I'm relearning what it means to be me," she said.

Michael Sieverts was another forced to recreate his sense of self. The fifty-eight-year-old former budget director for the National Science Foundation had spent a few weeks recovering from his Covid infection. He thought he was healthy again. But one day in early May 2020, he was digging up daylilies in his garden in Arlington, Virginia, when he felt the symptoms of a heart attack, including brutal chest pains and shortness of breath that, in his words, "put the SOB in SOB." One surprising symptom was the way in which he could stare at an email, knowing what the response ought to be, but not having the wherewithal to transfer the thought into written word. "I wanted to forward the note to my former self and have him write the response," Sieverts said. Eighteen months into the illness, he hadn't fulfilled his active retirement plans of becoming a yoga teacher or a ski instructor. Given his ongoing chronic illness and knowing what he knew about the complexity of funding major scientific breakthroughs, he was matter-of-fact in his tone with me. He knew he probably had a permanent disability.

Forging a life through disability was nothing new for Clare Daly, thirty-eight, the chief product officer at a tech startup in London. She had a master's degree in computer science and, before contracting Covid-19, was accustomed to working through complex problems. Daly had been diagnosed with myalgic encephalomyelitis when she was ten years old, which caused her body to recover poorly from viral illnesses. So, when she fell ill with Covid in December 2020, she knew how her story would unfold. "I told my boss immediately to find a replacement for me," she said. "And I spent the next month grieving for everything I would likely lose over the next year or so." Nearly six months after she caught Covid, she planned her whole week around voting by mail in London's May 2021 mayoral elections. It was a five-minute routine task that ate up days' worth of brain function.

"I noticed every tiny difference in phrasing between each vote as the cognitive load was excruciating," she said.

Losing brain function and the ability to comprehend sentences also struck at the core of Yvette Walker, a fifty-one-year-old writer in New Zealand. She was working on a book manuscript when she contracted Covid-19 in early 2020. For the first few months, she felt like the illness was an invisible gorilla that would throw her to the ground every day. "It felt like I had eight tropical diseases at once," she said. Eighteen months in, she hadn't managed to write any more of her book, or even finish reading a novel. Her brain MRI had come up clear, but her neurologist explained to her it didn't mean the virus hadn't affected her brain. By the fall of 2021, she was seeking out a neuropsychologist for more tests. "From my vantage point on the couch, I can see one of my many bookcases," she told me. "I find myself staring at that particular bookcase a lot. I think it's an unconscious yearning for reading and writing. I lean towards the bookshelf, hoping to return to my former life somehow, but I can't get through. It's maddening. I despair."

Disease can be devastating in how it can appear to target us in the areas where we're most passionate, cutting into the joys that make us feel most alive. Just as the virus dismantled Walker's love of the written word, it homed in on Kimberly Shay's taste buds. The forty-seven-year-old nurse from Albuquerque, New Mexico, had achieved nearly a sommelier level in wine tasting, but after losing her sense of smell and taste, could no longer discern the differences between flavors.

It performed a similar malice to Courtney Garvin, a singer and guitarist from Los Angeles. Her voice went silent. After seventeen months of illness, she still found it hard to speak, let alone sing. In August 2021, she remained bedbound most of the time and needed a wheelchair to get around. She didn't expect to ever play a concert again or brave the rigors of touring to perform on the road.

And for Molly Adams, Covid broke into her deep passion for birding, conservation, and wildlife. She had worked full-time in advocacy and outreach for the New York City Audubon Society and founded the Feminist Bird Club, roles that included taking groups on bird walks. But just looking through binoculars made Adams feel dizzy, listening to bird calls resulted in sensory overwhelm, and standing for more than twenty minutes triggered racing heart symptoms that could lead to fainting. Sending a fundraising email was impossible. Six months after first falling ill in February 2021, the conservationist couldn't work or participate in many of the activities that brought her joy and independence. "But I'm happy just to be here," Adams said.

Among those I connected with, that loss of connection to work or hobbies or loved ones forced a reassessment of what's actually possible in life.

"I was always outside with friends and was a very active person with a lot of hobbies," Bahtiyar Bozkurt, a thirty-seven-year-old engineer in Munich, Germany, told me. He had been planning a week-long hike with his girlfriend in Turkey, which became impossible after his illness onset in November 2020. "Now I'm bedridden and can't join anything. I'm unable to work," he said. "I loved to work, solve problems, and be creative. My concept as a human being is totally broken."

Cali Wilson was similarly cut off from the basic activities of daily living. The twenty-five-year-old anthropologist from Utah woke up on a particularly warm day in March 2020 and her life completely changed. Her breathing was labored, but she planned to take her dog for a walk after doing a few chores. When she returned from taking out the trash, however, she couldn't breathe or think, and felt like she was going to pass out. She spent the next eight months fighting for her life, and the next eighteen trapped in her small apartment.

"I never took my dog for that walk. I still haven't been able to," she told me. "That was my last day of freedom."

Marie, a twenty-six-year-old hacker in Silicon Valley, had intermittent fevers for weeks beginning in late February 2020, and was continually surprised by how "post-exertional malaise" would make her crash for days each time over the next year and a half when she went to the gym and tried to reclaim her old vigor.

That concept of post-exertional malaise is among the most important in this book, and perhaps the central theme marking Long Covid as a distinct health condition. It describes a physiological shutdown often following what could be even a minimal physical exertion or mental stressor. It becomes impossible to push through and accomplish daily tasks when your body crashes so completely and needs days to recover.

"I remember thinking that in a twisted way, I would almost rather be dying, because maybe then someone would finally listen," Marie wrote to me. "Maybe someone would investigate and find out what was wrong with me, instead of rolling their eyes and diagnosing me with Just Anxiety (Female Subtype)."

Rabia Jaffer, a teacher from Toronto, was stuck in Cape Town, South Africa for a year following her Covid infection, too sick to make the flight home. She fell ill in mid-March 2020, and each time she attempted to fly, she was thwarted by heart issues, collapsed lungs, or a frozen shoulder. Her recovery was all the more difficult due to the specter of closing borders, canceled flights, expiring visas, lapsing medical coverage, months-long lockdowns, and not knowing anyone in the city where she stayed for a year.

Marjorie Roberts, a life coach from Georgia, reported losing seven teeth due to dental problems brought on by Covid-19. Tooth loss came up again and again in online support groups, not at all uncommon among the seemingly unpredictable outcomes of the virus throughout the body.

Dani Mortell had summited Mt. Whitney, the tallest peak in the contiguous U.S., in October 2019. By October 2020, five months after her Covid diagnosis, she was struggling to walk two neighborhood blocks, and some days was completely bedridden.

Kimberley Grant, a social worker in Aberdeenshire, Scotland, went from being "fit and healthy to not being able to climb a set of stairs without feeling awful."

For Alexis Misko, an occupational therapist from Columbus, Ohio, that same failure to recover from minor activity became one of the most prominent aspects of life after the infection. "This is the worst symptom for me, even worse than the fatigue, because it makes me feel like I have no control over my own body, like I am in prison or walking on eggshells just to exist," she told me. "Sometimes my mom texts me because she is afraid I am lonely. She thinks that I am lonely for people, but I am lonely for life itself, because of post-exertional malaise." Her husband had gotten sick at the same time, and while he had a minor case, Misko's had been more severe, and much more chronic.

Esther La Russa, a cashier from Illinois, got sick on May 20, 2020, and said that while she had not required intubation, the virus nearly killed her. La Russa would lose the ability to stay awake or move her body after house cleaning or watching her toddler for twenty minutes. She and her partner had to forgo their wedding plans. Both could no longer work, needing help cleaning dishes, caring for their toddler, and getting rides to doctor's appointments. But their relationship deepened as they learned who they could trust and who would believe their new disability. "It helped our spiritual and emotional growth, though it was like aging ten years in eighteen months," she said.

Felipe Andrés Araya Casanova, a thirty-two-year-old government worker living near the coast in Chile's Iquique province, caught the virus in April 2020 and still felt a sore throat and stomach pains eighteen months later.

In the aftermath of catching Covid during the first winter wave, Eva Amat, a fifty-one-year-old secretary in Barcelona, suddenly found that while reading, there were words she could no longer understand, and that she was getting lost just walking in the streets where she lived. Seven months later, she felt she might be recovering bit by bit.

Joni Savolainen, a thirty-five-year-old man in Finland, was infected during the first wave along with his girlfriend, and reported feeling thirty to fifty different symptoms, including joint pain in his elbow that made it impossible to do his job working in IT.

Jenna, a young woman working as a product manager for a streaming service (and who wanted to keep her last name private), was infected early in the pandemic while living in Manhattan's Tribeca neighborhood. She spent her first seven weeks of illness alone in her apartment, after being told she was still contagious if she still had symptoms. She was so severely ill she could barely lift herself. She eventually drove to Virginia to stay with her parents for support. She was worried her life-long goal of attending business school was slipping out of reach, when at age twenty-four it took her a whole minute to figure out 2 + 6 and she "botched" her GMAT exam, required for entry into MBA programs. "No one reaches out anymore since they can't see us long haulers, since we stay at home sick and aren't visible to the world," she said. "I am one hundred percent missing out on my twenties and disappointed about it."

Jenna's overwhelming sense of isolation and loneliness were part of a common thread tying together the lives of many long haulers who shared their stories with me. Their suffering yanked them out of their usual jobs, routines, and friend circles. With their normal support systems faltering, they gravitated toward online peer support groups, gathering virtually with whoever they could find who was engaged in the same personal struggle and with who they shared the same new unwanted identity.

Enya Vermeyen, a mathematics teacher in Belgium, was one of those who found solace in connecting with other patients online. "There was nobody else to tell us how this would go and how long we would be stuck with long-term symptoms," she said.

Deborah Lee, a twenty-six-year-old consultant from Washington, D.C., also found support in patient groups on Reddit, Facebook, and Slack, which were far more effective in educating her about her new illness than any clinic she visited. "We were validated by each other when we were gaslit by our doctors," she said. But online peer support is far from a cure, and it can't patch over the dramatic effects an untreatable chronic disease can have on a life. "I was at the top of my career and Long Covid stole that from me. I was too dizzy and weak to sit up at a desk to take my Zoom meetings," she explained. "I got a new job and I felt like a failure. I also lost a relationship because my partner didn't know how to handle me suddenly being disabled and in despair."

Online support groups provide at least some sense of solidarity for people with the means. But in prison, getting basic healthcare or rudimentary tidbits of news is challenging. James McMillan, incarcerated at Bradshaw State Jail in Henderson, Texas, likely caught the virus in June 2020 when it was rampant in the facility during the first wave of the pandemic. Due to a shortage of tests in the facility, McMillan never had an opportunity to be tested but was isolated in a single-man quarantine cell while suffering back pain, respiratory symptoms, and headaches, he told me. At thirty-one years old, McMillan was serving his first year of an eight-year sentence and had, in part, been passing the time by working out two to three hours per day, an exercise regimen he'd maintained for the better part of a decade. But for the next year, he found he couldn't work out at all. Eventually he worked his way up to short, light workouts that were still a fraction of what he was used to. "I'm not even able to bring my body to a level of soreness," he said. "I can't even find energy to blow off steam. It's not just a fucking cold. It's more than that."

And just as McMillan had to fend for himself with infuriating post-viral symptoms in prison, Amanda Finley experienced her own fallout while frequently being unsure if she'd be able to have a roof over her head at night. The archeologist and single mom from Kansas City, Missouri, started a Facebook support group early in the pandemic that would eventually attract more than fourteen thousand members. She focused on trying to provide mutual aid, or small direct payments to individuals in dire need of medicine or shelter. Finley, who had asthma prior to getting Covid in March 2020, lost her apartment while contending with months of her disabling aftermath. Homeless, she temporarily moved in with a family from her church and then subsequently split her time between living in hotel rooms and sleeping in a tent at a national park campground. As the weather was growing colder in October 2021 and the tent was her only shelter, she sobbed as she spoke to me. She had dedicated herself to helping other long haulers, and through her group had gotten close with a number of people who had died from Covid complications, despite trying to rally support for them. At her chilly campsite, she feared that she too was on the verge of becoming another casualty of the pandemic.

Álvaro Rial, thirty, was infected during a trip to the U.S. in March, before returning home to northwest Spain. He told me the illness had contributed to his marriage ending in divorce, and seventeen months later he still had not resumed working again.

ONE VIRUS, MULTIPLE DISEASES

Beyond the primary acute disease of Covid-19, the SARS-CoV-2 virus can cause other conditions.

In children, the virus can cause a rare condition known as multisystem inflammatory syndrome, or MIS-C, which resembles the symptoms of Kawasaki disease, a rare condition originally described in Japan in the 1960s that causes inflammation in the blood vessel walls of children. While the symptoms can be severe, most patients recover within a few weeks with treatment. Those who go on to develop MIS-C tend to start by seemingly recovering from a mild or asymptomatic case of Covid only to have an inflammatory attack weeks later. The abnormal immune response can cause problems for them in their heart, lungs, kidneys, brain, skin, and gastrointestinal organs and land them in the hospital in need of critical care. By April 2022, MIS-C had appeared in about 7,880 U.S. pediatric Covid cases, killing 66. A similar inflammatory syndrome, MIS-A, can occur in adults.

Scientists observe that, under the umbrella of post-Covid conditions, the most obvious problem from a severe respiratory infection like Covid is the likelihood of causing permanent damage to the lungs, heart, and other organs. And beyond the cases of visible organ damage, many patients with acute Covid who were placed on ventilator go on to develop post-intensive care syndrome, or PICS, a well-characterized condition with physical, mental, and emotional effects. In recent decades, with more hospitalized patients surviving critical illness, PICS has become more common in those who recover from stays in intensive care units. Patients have muscle weakness, difficulty breathing, and decreased mobility. Moreover, they experience cognitive symptoms including decreased memory and poor concentration that can last for weeks, months, or years. And the syndrome's emotional symptoms include post-traumatic stress disorder, depression, and clinical anxiety.

Not surprisingly, PICS affects vulnerable minority populations in greater numbers than their non-minority equivalents. This fact is the culmination of a long list of systemic healthcare injustices—failures even—that were all present prior to the pandemic itself. Specifically in relation to PICS, however, people in vulnerable communities, including Black and Latino people, who disproportionately receive lower quality insurance coverage such as Medicaid, have less access to post-acute hospital care. People with less structured post-ICU care and rehab have worse long-term health outcomes. Even in situations where Black and Latino people are discharged into post-hospital settings, they are, on average, sent to lesser quality or inadequate rehabilitation facilities, compounding the health disparities even further.

The chronic consequences for which many doctors were much less prepared, however, were what came to be called Long Covid. As the pandemic progressed, hundreds of studies showed that multisystem illness could linger for weeks, months, or longer in an estimated 10 percent to 30 percent of those infected, or even more. It often occurred in patients with milder symptoms who were not hospitalized and wasn't related to the severity of the initial illness. Their bodies ostensibly recovered from the short-term acute symptoms—chills, fever, cough, loss of smell—only to be engulfed by fatigue, brain fog, and as many as two hundred other distinct symptoms. These patients frequently experience dysautonomia, a disruption of the autonomic nervous system, which is responsible for governing unconscious functions of the body such as heartbeat and digestion. They also commonly developed exercise intolerance, which turned even simple, everyday activities into Herculean tasks. Long Covid became—by far—the largest category of post-acute illness, casting a shadow over the lives of survivors, with eerie portents for the economic future of an increasing size of the working age population who'd come down with it through no fault of their own.

The Covid death rate in most developed countries falls within a range of a few percentage points, with a U.S. case fatality rate of 1.2 percent, according to Johns Hopkins University. So even taking a more conservative assumption—with 10 percent of infections leading to long-term symptoms—the risk of developing a significant post-Covid condition is eight times more likely than death. And many who develop profound life-altering disabilities report they can sometimes feel as though they've entered a state worse than death. Chronic effects are overwhelmingly the most concerning aspect of catching the virus for any particular individual, particularly the young and otherwise healthy, who are at the prime of their working years and who make up the heart of the labor force. Vaccines, with their low risk of adverse events, are vastly preferable to months or years of downstream effects from the virus.

But throughout much of the first two years of the pandemic, public health messaging often failed to frame Covid risk in terms of the possibility of long-term disability, a narrative baked into the earliest days of the outbreak.

For instance, the World Health Organization's report in February 2020 had put the median recovery time for mild cases at two weeks and for more severe or critical cases at three to six weeks. With hospitals and public health systems overwhelmed, the illness was first characterized and researched by patients who found each other online when the effects of the virus didn't resolve the way authorities had originally told them it would. Many had no medical degree or academic specialization in infectious disease or immunology. What they had was a suffering human body, the consciousness to describe it, and technological tools to form a global collective of citizen scientists called to action.

A NEW IDENTITY

One of those citizen scientists was Amy Watson, a forty-seven-year-old preschool teacher in Portland, Oregon, who fell sick on March 15, 2020, with a dry cough and flu-like symptoms. With Covid testing scarce and being saved for hospitalized patients, she followed the official advice and hunkered down to ride out the illness in isolation. She rested at home for weeks, hoping in vain to recover. At last, she threw on her lucky long haul trucker hat to cover up her unwashed hair and drove to get a Covid test, which came out positive.

She posted a selfie in the trucker hat on April 11, later declaring herself a Covid-19 "long hauler."

She founded the private Facebook group Long Haul Covid Fighters to support others who caught the virus and were plagued with "long haul" symptoms. It boomed in popularity, attracting thousands of members.

"Our somewhat goofy group name comes from my favorite trucker cap I wore when I got my first COVID test at a drive-up site," she explained in a post. "I'm starting to think maybe it's not so lucky..."

Due to Watson's group, the term *long hauler* exploded into the larger cultural dialogue of our time. By the following January, in less than a year, it was memorialized in the Merriam-Webster dictionary—alongside words such as *second gentleman*—as a new essential part of the English language.

Folksy and gritty, grim and yet forward-looking, it described the collective fate of millions during the greatest year of global upheaval in the twenty-first century.

Chapter 3

A GROUNDSWELL OF PATIENT ACTIVISM

Fiona Lowenstein, a twenty-six-year-old freelance writer living in New York City, was young and healthy, the living portrait of the person we'd have originally expected to be able to fight off the coronavirus quickly. Lowenstein exercised six times a week, didn't have asthma or any pre-existing conditions, and didn't smoke cigarettes. For someone with that profile, falling ill might mean symptoms for a couple weeks before moving on with life, or so the story went. Recovery, however, did not come quickly.

But much of Lowenstein's life experience made the young writer uniquely poised to speak on behalf of people whose bodies didn't exactly respond or behave the way experts predicted. Identifying as gender non-binary helped form the lens through which she viewed the world, including the medical community.

Lowenstein was born into a radical family and shaped by a rich set of influences. Barbara Seaman, a leader in the women's health movement famed for writings questioning the safety and efficacy of birth control, was like a "surrogate grandma" growing up. Seaman had campaigned on behalf of patients for side-effects' warnings to be inserted into birth control packages, and she had been memorably photographed waving a contraceptive on her finger while speaking at a news conference. The activist gave the young Lowenstein readings and took them to documentary film screenings and events featuring figures like feminist icon Gloria Steinem.

As a history major at Yale, Lowenstein prospered in classes on civil rights movements, activism, and women's liberation. They were editor-in-chief of the feminist publication, *Broad Recognition*, a platform they used to highlight hot-button social issues on campus, including sexual assault. They enrolled in a formative seminar under the legendary Washington reporter Bob Woodward, which shaped their thinking on investigative journalism.

After graduating, they spent a year working in the book publishing industry but quit at the prospect of years of ladder-climbing before having a chance at meaningful work. Feeling depressed and alone, they sought purpose in building a community with others who shared their ideals, not unlike those they had grown close with at the Yale Women's Center. "I just felt like, why not just start something that I actually want to attend?" they explained to me.

In March 2018, Lowenstein founded Body Politic, which called itself a queer feminist wellness collective and media company focused on staging events and dialogues at the intersection of health, wellness, and social justice. The group's name references a concept in political philosophy dating at least to Plato's *The Republic*, in which a political entity such as a city or state is imbued with the characteristics of a body. A king or sovereign acts as the brain, and the mass of citizens therefore as the organs and limbs. In Plato's analogy between the state and the soul, he argues that our society can be at equilibrium, he argues, if we, ourselves, can find the balance inwardly.

Finding that type of wellness is one thing if you're born into a stable social position. But many marginalized groups don't have that privilege. Lowenstein adapted the term *body politic* to build a space supporting and amplifying voices often sidelined or excluded from mainstream conversations about the politics of health.

"You're born into a body. The world treats that body a certain way. You don't always have a choice in how the world is interacting with you," Lowenstein explained. "I think that's especially the case for women and [people of color], for LGBTQ+ people, disabled and fat people."

The group was tapping into uniquely democratic ideas about individuals' capacity to express their own innate right for self-determination. It showcased a faith that the energy of change can flow powerfully from those marginalized at the fringes of society, whose voices are often drowned out by elites.

"I wanted wellness offerings that were not filled with straight, wealthy white women of a certain body type," Lowenstein said. "I wanted wellness offerings that were explicitly political and recognize the intersections of health and social justice."

Body Politic's first event only attracted about a dozen attendees. But the next one, called Body Talk, which featured people standing up to tell short stories, sold out. Panels followed on topics such as size and inclusivity in fitness, or sexuality and movement. They started partnering with more established publications. "*Bon Appetit* came and covered one of our events," Lowenstein said. "By the fall of 2019, I felt like we were starting to get some serious traction that could result in it getting funded or something, so that was actually my goal going into 2020."

The organization would take off in 2020, just a little differently. On March 10, a friend and fellow Body Politic co-organizer, Sabrina Bleich, visited Lowenstein's apartment for what each thought was the organization's final in-person planning meeting before New York's Covid-19 lockdown kicked in. Bleich also unknowingly brought over the virus.

The two friends fell ill.

Soon after, Lowenstein developed a fever and headache, and within two days they awoke in the middle of the night vomiting. Their shortness of breath had become so severe that they were gasping for air if they tried to speak a few words or walk to the bathroom. Their partner called the hospital and they headed to the emergency room Monday morning, where Lowenstein, at only twenty-six years old, finally found some relief after being given an oxygen tube.

"I got a look 'inside,' and received vital information that other people could use, both in terms of what was going on at the hospital but also everything that led up to that," Lowenstein said. "All of the calls to the department of health to try and get a test and being told I couldn't, and then my partner was also infected, as was the person who infected me, and watching their journeys trying to get care and trying to get tests." While many were sheltered at home anxiously following international news in the early days of the pandemic, Lowenstein had been thrust into a role of living the story.

Discharged on Wednesday, March 18, Lowenstein wrote several social media posts to explain what happened, and to let anyone with recent direct contact know they might have been exposed to the virus.

They reached out to a friend working as a fact-checker on the *New York Times* opinion page, on the off-chance that the paper of record might publish a first-person hospitalization account.

Editors agreed to it, and Lowenstein cranked out the piece in a couple hours on Friday morning. It went up the following Monday. The op-ed recounted how the coronavirus had landed the young writer in the hospital on a breathing tube and warned millennials to take the virus seriously.

In the weeks that followed, however, they were surprised to find that many symptoms didn't go away after leaving the hospital. Lowenstein started a group chat through WhatsApp where members could swap harrowing stories of Covid-19 and share tips for reckoning with symptoms. One person in the group, for instance, reported a fever of 100 degrees for four weeks. The group was originally intended as a small club, but friends kept adding other sick friends and the format quickly became untenable, with new messages pinging every second.

Lowenstein had a friend working who coached them through creating a group on Slack, an app favored by large organizations trying to keep all their internal communications in one place, with channels curated by topic.

Lowenstein pitched a follow-up op-ed to the *Times* to describe the ongoing multisystem symptoms experienced by non-hospitalized patients, which hadn't been reported anywhere in the media. This second piece, published on April 13, 2020, detailed how many of their Covid-19 symptoms weren't going away and how, in the weeks after diagnosis, they had gastrointestinal issues, loss of smell, fatigue, headaches, congestion, a sore throat, difficulty concentrating, and short-term memory loss.

No one expected to find so many desperate people exasperated by the same symptoms.

"Over the past two weeks, people from all over the world have joined," the article explained. "And one of the most common topics of discussion has been how complicated the recovery process has been—more complicated than is widely realized."

The stories other patients shared in the group showed that whole lives and families were being upended when sufferers weren't healthy enough to return to work after quarantining.

"Employers will need to reconsider expectations of Covid-19 survivors, and we can expect disability law to be tested," Lowenstein wrote. "A wave of chronically ill and slow-healing survivors is an inevitability we can and must prepare ourselves for."

The piece exploded with interest.

On one hand, it was a relief to know that the argument had validity and people as far as London or Italy wanted to join in discussing their long-term symptoms, asking for admission to the support group via the link on Body Politic's website. But on the other hand, what had begun as a volunteer-run startup hosting panel discussions in New York City transformed, virtually overnight, into the hub of a global patient movement.

"Within twenty-four hours of being published, over 2,000 people had signed up to join the support group. I remember just sitting there watching the Google form populate, literally one response every second," Lowenstein observed. With each snap of the finger there was a new member.

The torrent of new members desperately fumbling through the confusing aftermath of Covid was daunting. And the lack of answers from doctors or public health officials was terrifying.

"It also made me feel like what the fuck is going on that we haven't been acknowledging this at all and I had no idea this was happening to people? There's clearly so many people out there who need support," Lowenstein commented. "How am I gonna support all these people because I'm already running a volunteer organization? Most of the people on the team were dealing with their own pandemic-related crises because we're all in New York

City and it was March. Half of us were sick with Covid. So that was very stressful."

The concept of reframing the "body politic" would also come to act as a metaphor for notions about how vital information about the long-term effects of Covid-19 would first come from regular citizen scientists rather than the political and medical establishment.

"The people who are actually living the illness themselves are sometimes the only people who can speak to what the new symptoms are, and we saw everything," Lowenstein told me. "All the symptoms—Covid toes, hair loss, menstrual issues, neurological issues—all those symptoms that weren't as widely discussed were coming up in the group for months before they were widely talked about."

This was real-time data. A heartbeat at the center of the pandemic, a harbinger of what was to come.

A PARALLEL MYSTERY

One key member of the Body Politic support group didn't have Covid at all. A Colorado-based patient advocate and musician, Alison Sbrana had fallen ill with mononucleosis in 2014 as a college junior studying classical flute. Her first symptoms surfaced as a horrible neck pain while she was performing in the orchestra pit during the opera *Cendrillon*, the French rendition of the Cinderella story. It was the first sign she had mono, a condition sometimes called the "kissing disease," which is caused by the Epstein-Barr virus and can often be spread through saliva.

The common condition is almost something of a rite of passage among high school and college kids. Patients experience severe fatigue and swollen glands and need to rest, but it tends to clear up in four to six weeks. While most people make a full recovery, some studies suggest that as many as 10 percent with mono develop long-term symptoms lasting for more than six months. Sbrana was one of the unlucky ones.

"My life has never been the same since that day," she told me, recounting a story she felt was a cautionary tale for anyone dealing with the aftermath of a virus. "I declined over my first five years of illness to the point of being on disability, of requiring a wheelchair or mobility scooter, of basically being housebound."

Her fatigue, and her body's viral response, never seemed to subside in the way they normally should. Doctors diagnosed her with mast cell activation syndrome (MCAS), a condition in which mast cells, a type of immune cell responsible for triggering allergic reactions, become overactive and repeatedly trigger anaphylactic responses such as hives, swelling, and difficulty breathing.

About six months later, in early 2015, a neurologist diagnosed Sbrana with postural orthostatic tachycardia syndrome, otherwise known as POTS, in which the heart rate skyrockets upon standing up, or even sitting up or turning over in bed; such is its scope that it can lead to extreme dizziness or even fainting. The specialist originally told her she could expect to recover within three to five years, but her health trended downward rather than upward. As is common with complex chronic illnesses, she was thrown into a long and tangled journey through the medical system.

After graduating, Sbrana was capable of working for a year as a care coordinator for the state of Colorado. She helped patients with complex chronic diseases navigate Medicaid and health insurance systems, a role that tapped into her hard-won expertise from her own life. But her health continued to decline, and when she could no longer work full time, she eventually needed to go on Social Security disability. In 2018, four years after mono had originally struck during that fateful opera performance at Colorado State, she was diagnosed with myalgic encephalomyelitis (ME), also called chronic fatigue syndrome (CFS), just as I had been more than a decade before. The disease's Latin scientific name refers to a "muscle pain-related brain and spinal cord inflammation," stemming from a theory, yet to be fully proven, that it is caused by inflammation. The symptoms are generally characterized by extreme fatigue, pain, sleep disturbances, disabling sensory overstimulation, and an inability to recover from exertion.

Each of her complex overlapping conditions—MCAS, POTS, and ME/CFS—are often associated with a viral infection that either persists or triggers debilitating reactions in the body for years or even decades after. While each of these diagnoses suffer from a lack of research, their effect on the population is broad. Even prior to the pandemic, more than 1 million Americans were believed to have each of them, with women more than twice as likely as men.

Around the four-year mark, in 2018, Sbrana stumbled upon a post in Reddit's CFS section highlighting a rare opportunity to enroll as one of forty test subjects in the National Institutes of Health's intramural study of post-infectious ME/CFS, a process that involved two trips to the federal agency's sprawling campus in Bethesda, Maryland, just outside the nation's capital.

The study, at the world's largest clinical research hospital, was submitting the cohort of post-infectious ME/CFS patients to the most in-depth testing ever attempted in the disease. The two-week battery of tests included X-rays, functional MRI scans, neuro-cognitive tests, a lumbar puncture, and extensive blood work. Because exercise intolerance is often considered the cardinal feature of ME/CFS, one of the key measures was a cardiopulmonary exercise test that involved riding an exercise bike while hooked up to machines that monitored her vital signs as well as how her body was processing energy. The fact that the test would cause a torturous crash was well known by both scientists and patient subjects. The point was to gather information about her body as she experienced post-exertional malaise, succumbing to a kind of full body exhaustion that can follow even the most basic activities such as taking a shower or climbing a set of stairs.

The term *malaise* doesn't begin to express what patients feel; some researchers prefer calling the phenomenon "post-exertional neuroimmune exhaustion." The physical and cognitive crash can last for days or weeks in some cases, feeling like a combination of the flu, a hangover, and a ten-mile run all at the same time. Importantly, post-exertional malaise isn't common in other diseases, while it's nearly universal in the ME/CFS experience. When the invisible red line between a regular facet of ordinary life and a devastating crash is fickle or even imperceptible, finding ways to pace oneself and manage activity was perhaps the best way of reckoning with a potential onslaught of symptoms around every corner. And understanding this phenomenon was therefore one of the most important ways toward identifying a biomarker that doctors and scientists could use to diagnose the befuddling disease quickly.

Such a biomarker wouldn't be a cure. But it might mean that those with debilitating post-viral conditions might at least be able to get a name for their malady in a matter of months rather than the years of false starts and dead ends that Sbrana, and many like her, go through. Moreover, it could transform the field of research on the disease, spring it from its sense of illegitimacy, and instigate a renaissance of clinical trials by finally giving drug makers a universal objective target to shoot at.

Sbrana's friends and family were particularly interested in hearing about a specific aspect of the study that involved overnight stays in a metabolic chamber, in which researchers carefully monitored everything that went in and out of her body. The NIH researchers controlled every aspect of her diet, passing food through slots in the room's windows so they could study how her body created energy. Pipes in the ceiling took in the carbon dioxide she breathed out. Her urine and stool samples were stored in a small refrigerator in the room for analysis.

The study's protocol called for patients to make a second trip to Bethesda for a similar gantlet of medical testing about a year after their first visit. Sbrana and her fiancé had scheduled their wedding for late 2019; all of the fanfare around the ceremony required particularly complex planning for a bride with a baffling set of conditions who was also participating in a cutting-edge scientific study. Overexerting herself could mean crashing for weeks. So, they slated their second NIH trip on their calendar to fall from late January into mid-February of 2020. That, they hoped, would ensure that she "would be strong enough, and have enough energy for the wedding, and have time to crash if it was really bad," Sbrana said.

That winter, when they arrived at the extensive medical complex, her husband grew apprehensive. Foreboding signs were posted around the clinical center, with screening questions asking if entrants to buildings had flu symptoms and whether they had traveled outside the country recently. It was the couple's first signs of Covid-19's gathering storm.

During downtime during those long days of observation, the then-twenty-six-year-old Sbrana followed reports of China locking down and the virus beginning to ravage Europe. While much of the narrative was about case counts, deaths, and lockdowns, she was haunted by what the survivors of the virus might face in the months or years after infection.

Few in the public were aware at the time of just how quickly science was moving to produce coronavirus vaccines. Before Sbrana had arrived at the NIH headquarters, scientists in China had already published the DNA sequence for SARS-CoV-2. Scientists at the NIH's Vaccine Research Center were working with the pharmaceutical company Moderna to customize a prototype mRNA vaccine for the coronavirus spike protein. They designed and manufactured the vaccine while Sbrana was there and launched the first phase of clinical trials the following month.

"They developed the vaccine for Covid that I eventually got in my arm in that same building while I was there and I didn't know about it," Sbrana said.

The breathtaking pace of innovation within that building would lead to one of the most important feats of science in twenty-first century history, eventually beating back the deadliest costs of the pandemic. But the view from the bedside of a disabled chronic illness patient was different. On the one hand, Sbrana felt it was deeply reassuring to finally be surrounded by some of the nation's finest doctors and scientists, who actually understood at least something about her disease. But on the other hand, in talking with the researchers and doctors examining her, it became clear that very similar disease processes would likely soon be at work in a portion of those infected with the novel coronavirus.

"I'm a post-viral case myself and I've just gone through all this post-infectious ME/CFS workup at NIH and I'm like, 'Oh my God,' this is about to be really bad," she told me. "This is going to cause so many cases like mine."

She and her husband left Bethesda on February 13, returning home to Fort Collins, Colorado, and she waited "for the first report" of Covid-19's long-term symptoms. It took two months, but it appeared, like clockwork.

When Lowenstein's *New York Times* story was published in mid-April, Sbrana campaigned to join the burgeoning Body Politic support group, explaining that although she didn't have Covid-19, she could guide patients along what she believed would be the inevitable permutations of this virus—and likely a great many types of infections—in the human body. It took a couple weeks of cajoling, but she was granted access to the Slack group, and given admin and moderator responsibilities.

"And so I just hit the ground running as much as a person with ME can, which is not running at all," she laughed.

Patients who didn't recover from Covid-19 in the weeks after infection poured into the support group complaining of symptoms they didn't understand. Sbrana knew from personal experience how post-viral syndromes develop, could easily infer what was likely to occur next for patients, and was ready to curate their conversations accordingly. The Slack group format made it easy to organize dedicated conversation channels by topic. She created a channel for dysautonomia, a condition characterized by dysregulation of the autonomic nervous system, which unconsciously controls basic functions such as heart rate or breathing. She also started a channel for allergies and immunology for those who exhibited signs of mast cell activation syndrome. Many of the discussions focused on fatigue and cognitive issues, or co-morbid conditions including POTS and MCAS. She moderated conversations in more than seventy channels, allowing patients to sort themselves into the conversational categories or buckets relevant to them, and answering questions as they were posed.

"I really did a lot of the work in the beginning to help make sure that patients were being supported, to educate them on how to talk to their doctor about medical terms and medical conditions that they needed to know," she told me. "It was about giving Body Politic support group members the support that I wish I had in month one of my illness."

She could directly apply her wisdom and experience coordinating care for complex patients to thousands who came to the group seeking answers.

"I felt like the last six years of my life had prepared me to respond in that moment to all of these people that were suffering," she said.

SORTING THE SIGNS

Hannah Davis, who was a thirty-two-year-old computer programmer and generative musician when she fell ill, would go on to become one of the most publicly visible people in the world addressing the suffering caused by Long Covid. She cultivated a position as the most prominent voice on social media who could translate the onslaught of new scientific information about the emerging condition. And she led calls for policies to address long haulers' medical, economic, and social needs. In spite of her new disability, and inspired by it, she consulted widely with government agencies about research priorities and was a frequent patient expert in media stories about the condition. But she entered the support group like anyone else: confused and seemingly alone.

Before the pandemic, Davis was known for her computer program that translated books into music, performing natural language processing on classic novels, seeking out the feelings and sentiments through the story, and then composing musical pieces following the same emotional or narrative arc. One of her projects, a symphony, had premiered at the Louvre in Paris.

Another one of her artificial intelligence art installations was called *The Laughing Room*, a collaboration with Jonny Sun that appeared at MIT. It invited participants to sit in a room that looked like a sitcom set with couches and comfy chairs, where they could crack jokes. The computer would run the laugh track when someone said something funny. Knowing that much of comedy can thrive on racist or sexist jokes, she had trained the AI using comedians who were female or persons of color, helping avoid the awkwardness of a room laughing at overtly offensive humor. Her work had earned her an invitation, just before the pandemic, to speak at the Library of Congress about efforts to root out bias in datasets.

Such professional experience in data set bias would prove useful for her when Davis got sick on March 25, 2020. The sensory data of her own experience diverged sharply from the narrative peddled by public health officials that first appeared in the media. The experience of Covid-19's long-term neurological effects was nothing if not a problem in biased sets of data. Few of the early reports mapped the vast gulf between severely ill hospitalized patients and those who got the sniffles for a couple days before rebounding back to their usual selves.

In literary terms, it was as though Covid-19 was presenting with two different plot lines or narrative arcs—those who were getting well as expected, and those who weren't. Davis and the thousands of voices in the group were mapping what felt like a completely separate trajectory.

For Davis' part, her first symptom was cognitive, rather than respiratory, appearing when she realized she couldn't read a basic message in a group text thread among friends.

"It wasn't until week three that I started getting nervous and that was about the same time when Fiona Lowenstein put out the op-ed in the *New York Times*, which had a link to the Slack group," Davis said. "I joined and just so many people were describing neurological symptoms, brain fog, cognitive dysfunction."

Davis had joined a number of online Covid-19 recovery groups but felt Body Politic shined above the rest. "The information is different. The organization is different. Those historical values informed everything in it. It made us not start from scratch," she said. "We didn't reinvent the wheel with health activism."

In the Slack group's #datanerds channel, she connected with Gina Assaf, a design strategist from Washington, D.C., who had earned her masters at Carnegie Mellon University focusing on human-computer interaction. Assaf's work in international development had her traveling abroad just about every month for projects in low-income nations. In her forties, she had no major pre-existing conditions and ran a few miles a few times a week. Assaf's respiratory symptoms first set in while running on March 20, 2020, when she felt as though her lungs didn't have enough capacity. Over the next week she ticked off many of the usual symptoms: fatigue, body ache, chills. Due to widespread testing shortages, Assaf wasn't able to get testing until her seventeenth day of illness, which came back negative. That's not uncommon. A majority of PCR tests come up negative by the three-week mark.

One of Assaf's best friends got sick and got better, but Assaf declined. She felt dizzy and exhausted. She was unnerved by unusual burning sensations. When she tried to stand up, her legs felt heavy, and she got dizzy. She was exhausted all the time.

"I talked to doctors, and I felt like they thought I was crazy," she told me. "I just wasn't getting better."

After Lowenstein's op-ed was published, Assaf piled into the Slack group with the thousands of others. She was amazed to find hundreds of others reporting similar stories, with symptoms doctors told them couldn't possibly be explained by Covid.

But, clearly, here they all were. She posed the question of creating a survey, which they built in two days using Google forms. Participants answered a long list of questions on topics including their testing status, the duration and range of their symptoms, their level of physical capacity or ability to work, and whether they were hospitalized (most weren't).

"There was nothing online for us, nothing, except for the article that Fiona wrote," Assaf said. "There wasn't anything about what this was—for people who were supposedly healthy. You heard a lot of the trauma cases, but there was nothing about people like us that weren't getting better. You felt the urgency."

Where were the doctors? Where was the medical information? Where were the experts?

Most participants found the survey through the Slack group, although they also posted the survey link to other social media sites, targeting those with Covid-19 symptoms extending beyond two weeks.

Lisa McCorkell, twenty-eight, who was finishing a master's degree in public policy from the University of California at Berkeley, offered to help analyze the incoming research data. In the ensuing months and years, she would use that background to serve as the group's point person in matters related to communicating the needs of patients to various U.S. government agencies.

Hannah Wei, a Canadian product consultant, was working on a symptom tracker. She believed she was likely infected on a flight from Taiwan to Vancouver in mid-March. Like Lowenstein, she had gone to the ER for shortness of breath and witnessed an entire health system in chaos firsthand.

"I remember sitting in the waiting room and there were other people just like me who were just as young, who were coughing their lungs out," she told me. Wei managed to get a lung X-ray, which showed viral abnormalities, but she was ultimately sent home without receiving a test, as all of that Vancouver hospital's tests had gone to Washington state, where the virus was rampant. Although she got nothing in the way of treatment, the experience was valuable for other reasons.

"I got to see what was really going on," she said. "I think that was the most important thing that left me with a really big impression on what's actually going on versus what was in the news."

Athena Akrami, a neuroscientist with a lab at University College London, joined the Slack group in the wake of her long haul symptoms. She noticed the survey, offered to help, and was given access to the private research channel. As a professor, she had experience with computation, machine learning, data analysis, and statistical modeling, and she could use her university position to seek ethical approval to ultimately publish the data. She jumped in for an intense week of data analysis processing the trove of information gathered in the survey.

Those five sick women—Davis, Assaf, and McCorkell in the U.S., Wei in Canada, and Akrami in the UK—formed the core of one of the most significant acts of patient activism in recent history. Their research clout would help guide decisions in national capitals the world over while also changing countless individual lives with the simple power of validation.

"The circumstances that brought us together in an informal setting were what made it unique," Assaf said. "One of the reasons why we were able to do this was we were a desperate group of people."

They had bootstrapped a multidisciplinary team, with each bringing a particular skill in research, design, policy, and analysis. The quintet was imbued with a collaborative spirit, making decisions together without ego or drama. Their methods adhered to the same standards and rigor of scientific research from a university lab. All of them were, in fact, trained researchers whose destinies just happened to converge during a particularly urgent time in the same virtual place. Now, certainly there are limitations to how representative a self-reported symptom survey shared on social media can be. But during the public health emergency, their patient-centric participatory model provided an insight about a new emerging disease, particularly among non-hospitalized patients, that could never have appeared so early, any other way. It may hold true that as new diseases rapidly emerge, where patients go, science and policy follow.

In a year in which nearly all human interaction shifted to be physically distant or remote, it was an essential service in first describing the collective plights of millions.

"It's really magical, and I don't understand how it happened," Davis said.

They uploaded the analysis on May 11, 2020, in the middle of lockdown. It was originally just shareable through Google Drive before they posted the study on the new website for what they deemed the Patient-Led Research Collaborative.

The survey generated 640 responses in twelve days. The data showed that 91 percent of patients in the group reported not recovering from the virus.

A FOUNDATIONAL CONTRIBUTION

Brain issues were one of the most notable results in the eight-week period the survey covered. Commonly, patients reported brain fog, concentration challenges, memory loss, seizures, dizziness, and balance problems. They reported neurological problems at a higher rate than they reported coughing or breathlessness. And almost two-thirds of those in the survey were between ages thirty and forty-nine. It was an early indication that younger people were vulnerable to longer term symptoms.

Collating the lived experiences of support group members this way also revealed another significant finding that exposed blind spots in the patchy system of testing, in which tests were either unavailable or unreliable or those of lower socioeconomic means had less access to healthcare services. Many people who had symptoms consistent with SARS-CoV-2 weren't able to get the validation of objective proof.

Just 23 percent of those who filled out the survey reported testing positive for the virus. Half couldn't get tests or were denied, and another quarter tested negative, partially because they were tested too late. The reported symptoms were consistent across the whole sample whether participants returned positive tests or not.

In the months afterward, the lack of positive test results would act to sort patients with long-term symptoms into a lesser tier, a constant burden that could potentially limit access to post-Covid clinics, hinder health or disability insurance approvals, hamper research efforts into long haulers' symptoms, or lay doubt as to whether their physical disease was believed at all. Often patients would struggle to receive a diagnosis from doctors based on symptoms alone.

Science writer Ed Yong spotted their signal within the noise, profiling members of the research team with a June 4, 2020 piece in *The Atlantic* with the headline "Covid-19 Can Last for Several Months." The story was a singular moment in elevating the plight of long haulers to international recognition, and part of a remarkable run of stories on all aspects of the Covid-19 crisis that would eventually win Yong the Pulitzer Prize for explanatory reporting the following year.

"When I created that report, I expected to get better," Assaf told me when I first talked to her in July 2021. She noted that she had originally believed that asking patients about even eight weeks of Covid-19 symptoms was too long a period. But more than sixteen months after the virus had announced itself by stopping her workout short, she was still feeling significant symptoms. She was seeing doctors to help with her memory and her heart and could work nowhere near the schedule she'd maintained before the pandemic.

Meanwhile in the spring of 2020, in the northern Italian region of Lombardy, an archeologist named Elisa Perego was beginning to deal with dozens of relapsing and recurring symptoms throughout her body in the wake of Covid-19. Perego had dealt with multiple chronic illnesses herself prior to contracting Covid. And as an academic, she had published papers on crisis and collapse in past societies, including work to understand disease and disability through studying ancient human remains.

"So at least, in part, I was conscious of what was happening to me," she wrote to me in an email in August 2021, explaining that seventeen months after she had first fallen ill, her ongoing symptoms, including issues with speaking and breathing, made it too difficult to speak over the phone.

On May 20, 2020, she tweeted an article about Covid from Italian newspaper *la Repubblica* along with the hashtag

#LongCovid to describe the dozens of symptoms she was feeling after the infection. She didn't realize she was coining the name of the new condition.

"As my own disease progressed, it was difficult to link my own lived experience with the partial representation of it in the early medical literature," she said. "This is why the online community was so important and validating."

The sense of validation quickly resonated with thousands. That English language social media hashtag #LongCovid would be used millions of times.

Patients discussed their persistent Covid symptoms under the Spanish language hashtag #covidpersistente. In German, they rallied around the term #mitcoronaleben, for "living with corona," and in French, the discussion centered around #apresjour20, or #apresj20, referring to symptoms continuing after day 20.

Claire Hastie, a corporate consultant in the UK, had become incapacitated by Covid, feeling pronounced pins and needles in her legs and intense pressure in her head that made her unable to call for help. After the terrifying first night of severe symptoms, she was surprised she woke up the next morning alive. "I said what I thought might be my last words to one of my sons who happened to pass by the next morning," she told me. She'd been used to cycling thirteen miles to work each day. But seven weeks after falling ill, she still needed to be cared for by her kids, who had to learn to cook and do household chores while sick themselves. "I had never set up a Facebook group before. I'm famously not very techie, but I pressed a few buttons in my ill haze." She launched the community that would come to be called Long Covid Support Group, using the term Perego had invented. Tens of thousands of people joined from 100 countries. The idea was snowballing.

"This is one reason why we say Long Covid is collectively made," Perego told me. "The hive mind and sharing of the community were instrumental in consolidating concepts of the disease, long duration, the presence of symptoms not reported in the early literature, and in breaking down concepts such as 'mild.'"

Long Covid is just as likely to stem from a mild case as it is from a severe case. And because mild cases are much more common, Long Covid therefore disproportionately occurs in mild cases. But the concept of mild can also have a different meaning in pandemic medicine than in common, colloquial usage. You could have the worst illness of your life, but unless it was bad enough to require hospitalization, it could still be considered mild. And for one in ten people, it can become chronic.

Patients launched support groups and advocacy campaigns in a growing list of countries. Juno Simorangkir launched a campaign in Indonesia. On July 8, 2020, the UK patient group LongCovidSOS posted a "Message in a Bottle" YouTube video, addressed to the WHO, which featured dozens with Long Covid holding handwritten signs indicating how long they'd been sick and what their most pernicious symptoms were. One woman peaked at "DAY 131: ALIVE BUT NOT LIVING." A nine-year-old boy wrote a sign in a green marker complaining of fatigue, brain fog, loss of appetite, nausea, and stiff limbs.

"Our numbers are growing, and we need to be taken seriously," the video's narrator said. "We need rehab, research, and recognition. We need to be believed, helped, treated with compassion, and supported by those around us. Please hear our SOS."

To reinforce the argument, two days later, a group of doctors in the UK with Long Covid symptoms published a *British Medical Journal* opinion piece arguing that the country's National Health Service wasn't including thousands of long haulers with symptoms beyond sixteen weeks in its Covid-19 narrative. It critiqued top-down approaches and highlighted the patient-led research emerging from Body Politic's Slack group as a model to follow. They called for acute Covid to be classified as a separate condition altogether from Long Covid, and for detailed epidemiological studies to gauge how common the longer version of the disease was.

INSTITUTIONS TAKE NOTE

That same week, during a virtual press conference about Covid-19 following the International AIDS Conference, Terri Wilder, a social worker and HIV activist from New York City, posed a question to Dr. Anthony Fauci, Director of the National Institute of Allergy and Infectious Diseases, about whether public officials were looking into the post-viral diseases long haulers were developing.

"If you look anecdotally," Fauci responded, "there is no question that there are a considerable number of individuals who have a post-viral syndrome that really in many respects can incapacitate them for weeks and weeks following so-called recovery and clearing of the virus."

He noted reading stories in social media groups for Covid-19 patients who reported not getting back to normal after a bout with the virus.

"They have things that are highly suggestive of myalgic encephalomyelitis and chronic fatigue syndrome—brain fog, fatigue, and difficulty in concentrating," he explained. "So this is something we really need to seriously look at because it very well might be a post-viral syndrome associated with Covid-19."

The LongCovidSOS group organized a virtual meeting with the WHO which included dozens of long haulers from around the world. For an hour and a half on Friday, August 21, 2020, patient representatives from the U.S., UK, Senegal, and South Africa shared their stories with WHO officials, including its head of clinical care and its technical lead for the Covid-19 response. Grounding the survivors' tales in empirical evidence, Davis presented the Patient-Led Research Collaborative's findings from the support group survey.

WHO Director-General Dr. Tedros Adhanom Ghebreyesus observed the meeting but didn't make it known that he was on the call until the end, surprising the guests by saying he had personally seen their "Message in a Bottle" video. He quoted part of a suffering British doctor's presentation back to the group, noting that "with patient-led research and patient-led activism, it appears that patients are writing the first textbook on Long Covid."

"All of us came to the understanding that we needed to roll out a second survey that would be more comprehensive, showing the symptoms that are even more complicated than the sixty in the first survey." Akrami said.

More and more long haulers completed an expanded survey with 260 different questions. And the patient-led team could see an increasingly detailed portrait of the disease further emerge, classifying symptoms into ten different organ systems.

They documented more than 200 symptoms in 3,762 long haulers from 56 countries over 7 months. Respondents reported "significant disability," with an average of fourteen symptoms well beyond breathlessness that were still ongoing six months after their initial infection. Fatigue was the most common at 78 percent. That was followed by post-exertional malaise, the primary marker for ME/CFS, at 72 percent and cognitive dysfunction at 55 percent.

Almost half said their symptoms were bad enough to require a reduced work schedule, and 22 percent could not work at all.

The results also showed that Long Covid was more common in women. Almost four out of five who completed the survey were women. Part of that could be attributed to general research trends that women are more likely to join support groups and to fill out surveys, but still, the results were consistent with an existing body of research that post-viral syndromes are more prevalent among women.

This time, with Akrami's sponsorship at University College London, the PLRC team wrote up the results in a paper for a medical journal.

In late December 2020, they uploaded the study to the preprint server medRxiv (pronounced "med archive"). The website, founded in 2019, is a joint project of scientists from the *BMJ*, Yale University, and Cold Spring Harbor Laboratory. It became one of the most common ways for researchers to post new studies during the pandemic. Papers posted there carried a disclaimer that they had yet to navigate the often lengthy and byzantine peer review process. But it was a helpful, life-saving innovation in the scientific process just in time for a global public health emergency. The website distributed vital information to the scientific community and the public more broadly, allowing new data to be disseminated and debated at the accelerated pace the crisis required.

Ultimately, the Patient-Led Research Collaborative study was published in the peer reviewed journal *EClinicalMedicine*, part of the family of medical journals run by The Lancet. But long before that, it became one of the most widely cited scientific papers of the pandemic, ranking in the top one-tenth of 1 percent of studies on the medRxiv server in terms of online attention.

Research generated by expert patients had become a foundational study into the widespread long-term suffering of which Covid-19 was actually capable.

Collaborating with British geography professor Felicity Callard, Perego published an article in the journal *Social Science & Medicine* that suggested "there are strong reasons to argue that Long Covid is the first illness to be made through patients finding one another on Twitter and other social media." The piece explained that Long Covid as a concept and disease entity "moved from patients, through various media, to formal clinical and policy channels in just a few months" and argued that informed and connected patients had "marshaled epistemic authority" in defining the new disease rather than relying on doctors and scientists.

SEIZING AUTHORITY

"As a disease recognized, named, and defined collectively by patients, Long Covid defies conventional categories of authority in medicine," Perego told me. "It shows to people that yes, patients *can*. We as patients have power, resources, and massive expertise. This has the potential to disrupt how biomedical knowledge is built and medicine should work."

In coining the term Long Covid and taking a role in driving the public debate, Perego benefitted from her prior knowledge of having lived with a chronic illness and being involved in disability activism. She visualized the global discussion as one in which the wisdom and power of people outside the established medical system had preempted the system itself.

"Covid patients' involvement is important because we know the condition. We have been through it as whole people, not just as a single organ, or body system. We have also known how the disease develops through time. It's a very dynamic disease with its own temporal development," Perego said.

That story was happening everywhere the virus touched. The WHO reported 1.65 million social media mentions of "Long Covid" during a three-month period in early 2021.

But given the life and death nature of the global emergency, bulky bureaucratic institutions couldn't adapt quickly in the moment to build a foundation that could address the long-term illness. For many crucial months that responsibility lay solely in the hands of patient communities, collecting and passing essential knowledge through informal networks.

"I gave so much blood, sweat, and tears to this group, especially in the early days because it was such a crucial time and no one else, like the government, was doing it," said Sbrana, the Colorado musician with ME/CFS. "I wish I had had this seven years ago and I maybe wouldn't be homebound having to use a wheelchair."

In addition to the post-viral diseases that Sbrana lived with, Body Politic's roots as a queer wellness group in New York helped center a set of cultural memories. This suggested emerging diseases, particularly those common in marginalized groups, didn't receive the resources and attention they required. The early history of the AIDS movement had been plagued by neglect, in part because HIV was perceived to be a gay disease rather than a mainstream problem.

Body Politic displayed its value of being "historically informed" prominently on its website. Sbrana's experiences in post-viral diseases fueled much of its work helping long haulers.

"When patients are not being believed by their doctors, this is not new. It's just that the problem is getting attention," she told me. "And so every meeting, I was that voice of saying, 'We need to recognize this is not new.'"

In the heady early days of the pandemic, lighting the spark of attention that Long Covid existed was the easy part. Working with scientists to launch effective research studies and supporting millions in the lengthy and unpredictable process of rehabilitation would be far more challenging.

Chapter 4

PATIENTS BECOME
THE EXPERTS

OUR WORD *PATIENT* COMES TO us from the Latin "patiens," meaning one who suffers. It calls to mind a passive recipient of care, one who is examined and subjected to, made to obey orders. The Patient-Led Research Collaborative reframed this relationship.

The team's research immediately became one of the most insightful studies of the pandemic. It captured an experience that couldn't yet be described via in-person hospital or laboratory settings. The surveys and support group were cited by the *New York Times*, *Vox*, MSNBC, CNN, the *Guardian*, NPR, *Buzzfeed*, and a list of other media organizations too numerous to count.

During an extended recovery, Fiona Lowenstein, Body Politic's founder, slept as long as possible each morning. Making breakfast and brushing teeth while seated still required building in time to rest after each basic task. That plodding routine made it possible to manage a few hours of computer work in the afternoon. And it helped in keeping up with a constant stream of interview requests and appearances on live TV news shows discussing personal symptoms and the hundreds of bizarre viral effects showing up in Body Politic support group members. But by late afternoon Lowenstein would start to crash and, on days of particularly intense light or sound sensitivity, had to lie still in the dark.

"I felt like after those first two op-eds I had to continue trying to write as much as possible in mainstream media publications, while also taking interviews to talk about what I was seeing," the young activist observed.

Lowenstein appreciated having a platform and being perceived as reputable, so wanted to use that position to benefit people with the new disease who weren't getting good care or even being believed by their doctors at all. "There were a lot of reasons why I was believed. I'm white, I went to Yale, and I'd had pieces in other publications like this before so I was seen as a legitimate source," they explained. "I felt like I had to bring what was going on in the group to the outside world because a lot of the people in the group were too sick or not in a position to go public with their story."

AGENCIES EXTEND A HAND

Various research groups from within the CDC started reaching out to AI artist Hannah Davis and the PLRC team in summer 2020, asking for feedback about post-Covid symptoms. One result of those conversations was a series of one-pagers from the agency about the symptoms, specifically listing post-exertional malaise as a feature of the illness, which had yet to be done.

NIH Director Francis Collins highlighted the research on his blog, calling it a "first-draft description of long COVID syndrome," and noting that "if even a small proportion of the vast numbers of people infected with Covid-19 develop Long Covid syndrome, it represents a significant public health concern." But with the snowballing interest from the public, researchers, and health agencies, there came sharp voices of dissent as well. As Covid became intensely politicized and anti-lockdown protesters gathered in city squares around the world, the act of sticking up for patients with long-term effects earned them criticism as being part of a pro-lockdown movement.

Older debates about post-viral illness surfaced as well. A resident psychiatrist from Canada, Dr. Jeremy Devine, penned a *Wall Street Journal* opinion piece criticizing the PLRC research for including patients in their survey who had not tested positive for the virus or who didn't have access to a test. He argued that it was a psychosomatic disorder driven by a false belief that one is ill and unlikely to recover—and that publicizing it would lead other "impressionable" patients to believe they had the condition too. Long Covid and symptoms following a coronavirus infection were "largely an invention of vocal patient activist groups," he argued. "Legitimizing it with generous funding risks worsening the symptoms the NIH is hoping to treat."

One stinging jab came from a well-known scientist who called the patient-led preprint "Mickey Mouse science at best." Seeing the ongoing suffering from thousands of support group members made it impossible for the team to just shake off those rebukes as the everyday jousting of professional scientific debate. It felt like a direct rejection of their lived experiences, of reality itself.

They still had each other, though they were spread across the globe from Oakland, California to London. Hannah Wei, the graphic designer among the group, drew up a mock logo for the PLRC with Mickey, Minnie, Donald Duck, and Goofy sitting under the bubble letters "Patient-Led Research Gals: Your Experts in 'Mickey Mouse Science.'" Below it, she wrote "As seen on…" and included the logos for the CDC, NIH, WHO, UK Parliament, and the UK's National Institute for Health Research.

The picture had their whole group in hysterics.

Hannah Davis presented patient-led research findings at the World Health Organization's private webinar organized by LongCovidSOS. She presented their research to the WHO multiple times, as well as CDC and NIH, and their findings were cited in the first mention of Long Covid in the British Parliament.

"It's possible that I would not be studying Long Covid—it's possible that a lot of people would not be studying Long Covid—if I didn't come across the patient-led survey and all the reaction to it," said Dr. Ziyad Al-Aly, Director of the Clinical Epidemiology Center, and Chief of the Research and Education Service at the VA St. Louis Health Care System, and an assistant professor of medicine at Washington University in St. Louis. "It's really possible that they changed the history of medicine."

Inspired by the patient-led example, he and his clinical epidemiology research lab set to work on a study that leveraged the full might of the U.S. Department of Veterans Affairs medical record system to get an all-encompassing view of Covid's post-acute "sequelae," or aftereffects, among veterans. "If Hannah Davis can do this, and she's sick and fatigued, and exhausted, why can't I work one or two more hours on a Saturday just to get this analysis done or to inch our paper toward completion?" Al-Aly pondered. His team's study was published a year into the pandemic in the influential journal *Nature*, the largest-ever controlled study of Long Covid patient records to that point. It compared more than 73,000 Covid survivors within the VA system to a much larger cohort of nearly five million individuals in the VA system who didn't get Covid. It found increased rates of cardiovascular complications, diabetes, and kidney disease, among other chronic conditions that some patients might end up living with for the rest of their lives. "What you're seeing now are the acute effects," he told me. "What we're seeing broadly as a society is the tip of the iceberg, compared with the death, disease, and disability that comes from Long Covid. What we see is really immense." Their data showed that even while many long haulers had symptoms of conditions that weren't well characterized, it was already clear that Covid's long-term burden on the health system would be measured across a spectrum of chronic diseases that are easily detectable.

The Patient-Led Research Collaborative had begun with no other goal than to support each other through the uncertainty of a deadly pandemic. But in a wider sweep of history, those with longer memories saw something more profound.

"They are amazing. They are heroes," Al-Aly said. "They are like the twenty-first century version of ACT UP and Larry Kramer. There are a lot of parallels."

Davis, born in the late 1980s, hadn't heard of Kramer.

Kramer, an Oscar-nominated screenwriter, playwright, and public health activist, had co-founded the Gay Men's Health Crisis in the early 1980s to address the issue of "gay cancer" that would eventually become known as AIDS. The GMHC became the largest organization serving men and women living with AIDS. In 1987, Kramer was also the spark that ignited into the AIDS Coalition to Unleash Power (ACT UP), a political direct-action organization devoted to ending the AIDS pandemic through medical research, treatments, and legislation. ACT UP's in-your-face approach for galvanizing public sentiment—including actions that disrupted operations on Wall Street and the Roman Catholic Church—set the standard for a generation of health activism. Kramer and ACT UP eventually won a supporter in the young director of the National Institute of Allergy and Infectious Diseases, Dr. Anthony Fauci.

The group's actions were memorably depicted in the 2012 documentary *How to Survive a Plague*, which Davis watched for inspiration on the Long Covid fight. As a quiet, understated computer programmer, she had a style that departed from the brash speechmaking and over-the-top theatrics of ACT UP. For instance, ACT UP had once unfurled a giant condom to cover anti-gay Sen. Jesse Helms' house with words explaining the pro-phylactic was to "stop unsafe politics." Davis resonated with a different type of activist energy, dedicated to full immersion in the data of her disease, digesting each new research paper with ardent zeal, and disseminating the summaries to her blossoming Twitter following. She saw an historical counterpart in one of the AIDS film's characters who did a 1980s version of the same. ACT UP's Treatment & Data Committee had run teach-ins to educate patients about the science. Self-empowerment helped them sur-vive when dealing with medical providers who, at the time, knew less about the virus than they did.

"I really related to the guy who went the research route and wanted to learn everything," she said. "There were those scenes with him, especially early on, especially before they were their own organization, just standing there in front of this crowd and reading the research papers. It's just like the analog version of what our channel does all the time."

There were major differences between 1980s HIV activists and Long Covid activists. Perhaps most noticeably, organizing street protests wasn't possible when patients were bedridden and when public health measures prohibited large gatherings. And most people believed they would get better, and many were recovering, albeit slowly. Yet technological advancement brought new tools: Facebook, Twitter, Reddit, Slack, and other online platforms meant that patient communities could self-generate just about anywhere.

Like Kramer, Davis was an activist with an uncompromising vision, holding researchers to the exacting standard patients needed in order to get their lives back.

"No matter what, there is going to be research done in these fields. It's just whether or not we're going to have a cure," she said. "When I was working on the research outcomes for the WHO, it felt obvious to me to put a cure down as an objective. But a lot of people don't think of it that way. They think of it as we find a medication that makes your life tolerable and you can function. I really hope that we find a cure for ME and Long Covid."

You'd think that ought to be the goal of any medical research.

"But no one is really thinking of that and that's what's bothering me," Davis said. "And that's what happened with HIV, right? I mean they stopped funneling money into a cure as soon as they had anti-retrovirals."

Those drugs, which stop HIV from replicating in patients, can only control the virus, making it possible to live with HIV, not eliminate it outright.

LEADING FROM WHERE YOU SIT...OR LIE

Claire Hastie, the founder of the UK's Long Covid Support group, hatched the idea for the WHO to convene a global conference on Long Covid, which was held in early December of 2020. The forum, in which the organization's director general delivered the opening remarks, released an agenda identifying research priorities for funders and researchers.

"It was very much with patients at the heart. Patients were presenting. They were co-chairing a session. It was designed with short sessions and breaks for patients and videos of patient stories in between," she said.

As a leader in a prominent global support group, Hastie became a regular representative at government meetings representing the patient voice.

"We've been kicking ass from beneath our duvets. We were literally bedridden," she explained. At each meeting she expressed how appreciative she was about the work the officials were doing, but was very direct in conveying how severe the situation was among the patients in the group. Lives were ravaged, there weren't adequate treatments, and urgent radical action was required. Patients didn't need to log their 'lingering symptoms' in an app. They needed a cure.

"I've met the Secretary of State for Health. I've been in bed with Matt Hancock," she laughed, referencing the British member of Parliament who had led the cabinet's health efforts from 2018 to 2021. "I've spoken quite frankly to some really senior people. It kind of helps that you don't really know who these people are, and I'm not the one to be intimidated anyway. They're all just little squares on a Zoom screen."

Even as the UK created Long Covid clinics across the National Health Service and began planning large-scale research studies, Hastie was adamant in pressing the case, detailing how those efforts were largely not making meaningful impacts in the regular lives of long haulers, and how a number of studies were counterproductive, failing to partner meaningfully with patients or relying on flawed assumptions about the severity of the underlying disease process.

"I've had to say it really forcefully," Hastie said. "I've given presentations to the NHS task force where they've emailed me afterwards and said, 'Oh my God, that was really shocking.' They're working their backsides off and I'm massively appreciate of that, but we've got to report back what we're learning. We've heard senior people say by email afterwards that it 'really shook us to the core.' But we've also had plenty of people, who work in senior positions, saying of the patient movement, that they've just never seen the like. And I guess that's because they weren't involved in the HIV days because that's similar."

Patients could lead from wherever they sat, whatever position they held, whether that meant having nothing more than a Twitter feed, or a seat in the highest corridors of power. Virginia Sen. Tim Kaine had served as governor of his state and been tapped as Hillary Clinton's vice-presidential running mate in 2016. He announced in March 2020 that he and his wife had acute Covid-19 symptoms and tested positive for antibodies two months later. But that hadn't been the end of his story as he revealed during a Senate health committee hearing the following spring.

"I have these weird neurological symptoms a year later. They're not debilitating, they're not painful. But they're weird," Kaine said during the hearing, in which the NIH's Dr. Anthony Fauci and CDC Director Rochelle Walensky testified. "It just shows how tricky this virus is, and it also suggests that the long-term consequence in our health system is probably a lot bigger than we're thinking of right now."

Kaine explained to *US News and World Report* that Covid had left him with a nerve-tingling feeling "literally 24/7," with which he felt like he'd just had five cups of coffee. Following the infection, he'd had intermittent rashes, and a "heating pad phenomenon" in which parts of his skin would run hot for no apparent reason. Although he wasn't suffering, he felt highlighting his own personal story was a way to help further policy and believed that he was the only senator to bring up the issue of long-term symptoms during a hearing, which he did on two occasions. On March 18, 2021, he made a point to use his time to ask Fauci about the NIH's plans to study Long Covid.

Fauci gave a detailed response and Kaine said he had found the answer satisfying, mostly because Fauci, as the face of the nation's pandemic response, had simply offered validation to sufferers. Kaine's objective was to draw out that basic message. "What I really wanted was anybody watching this hearing who has Long Covid symptoms to hear Dr. Fauci say: 'This is not imaginary, this is real.'"

Members of the Patient-Led Research Collaborative were invited to testify in front of the House Energy and Commerce Committee on April 28, 2021. The committee has oversight of the Department of Health and Human Services, as well as FDA, CDC, and NIH.

For her testimony, Lisa McCorkell, the PLRC public policy specialist, logged into the virtual meeting from home, which started off with the type of technical glitches that had come to characterize life on video calls during the pandemic.

"We just couldn't get the YouTube stream to work at all, and so for the first thirty minutes of the hearing, it was just like me, the other witnesses, and the Congress members just chit-chatting, which was so bizarre, because they are just co-workers," she said. Hearing them make small talk about the weather and their families, the little squares on the Zoom screen were less intimidating than if they'd been perched behind their dais in a capacious hearing room.

When the meeting did come to order, NIH Director Francis Collins opened his testimony by commenting that the hearing was the most well-attended in his recent memory.

In her late twenties, McCorkell was a year out of her public policy degree at University of California at Berkeley and was working as a policy analyst in the state of California's Supplemental Nutrition Assistance Program. "I never thought that I would testify in front of Congress on anything," she told me. "Like maybe for something bad." Of course, millions of people with a life-altering disease *is* bad, but McCorkell and her fellow patient researchers were highlighted as heroes. Members of Congress went out of their way to praise their work, probe more deeply into the science, and to validate sufferers, many of whom were their own family members or constituents who contacted their legislators calling for action.

"What I have found very impressive in the testimony today and in discussions with other people is the Patient-Led Research Collaborative," Michigan Rep. Debbie Dingell said during the hearing. "The U.S. has unmatched research infrastructure and we've started to advance patient-centered research through organizations like [the Patient-Centered Outcomes Research Institute], but I'm really impressed with the ability of patients to self-organize around a new condition like long haul Covid and to get your voices together and to be effective quickly. And I think that's really important—to get your results quickly into the medical literature."

She followed up with a question about how McCorkell's group would sync up with the NIH, to help maximize the return on the government's investment of taxpayer dollars. At that point, some 200 different researchers or institutions had submitted grant proposals to grab a piece of the $1.15 billion that had been set aside to research long-term effects of SARS-CoV-2. Although the patient research group had an inbox overflowing with requests to collaborate, McCorkell was concerned that the NIH would award grants to researchers who didn't have a history of studying the relevant diseases, who weren't centering patients, and who might design their studies in ways that didn't address the actual needs of those who were sick.

"Our worry is that not all of them are going to incorporate the patient voice," she said. "Not all of them are going to incorporate past research into post-viral illness like ME/CFS. Not all of them are going to incorporate ME/CFS patients. And these are very critical in order to actually create findings that are going to be useful for Long Covid patients."

In their view, one of the PLRC's biggest successes came on June 14, 2021, when the CDC released its interim guidelines for treating post-Covid conditions. The guidance offered detailed information on which tests doctors should perform. It incorporated much of the feedback the Body Politic and PLRC had given, particularly that objective lab findings shouldn't be the only measure to assess a patient's well-being, and a positive Covid test shouldn't be required in order for a patient to gain access to a post-Covid clinic. They felt the CDC had listened.

McCorkell told me she cried when she got the news.

And Alison Sbrana, seven years after a post-viral illness had forever altered her life in college, found that in a few places in the document it was almost as though the world's leading public health agency had copy and pasted sentences from what she had written to its researchers. Her comments laid out key details on the best practices for managing the condition, particularly with few good drugs available. While she could revel in the moment of personal redemption, she knew the tactical victory for Long Covid was just the latest step building on the work of thousands of patient advocates who had been virtually trying to break down the agency's door for decades.

"I felt bad because I was like, who am I to get these red-carpet opportunities to meet with CDC and NIH when I've hardly been doing this very long relative to all these [longtime ME/CFS activists]. This has been their life's goal and they've never been given the opportunities to make this amount of progress," Sbrana said. "It would be disrespectful of all of those advocates who came before us, to not acknowledge all the work that they've done and to not build off of what they have done."

AN OPENING FOR A FORGOTTEN ILLNESS

Before Covid-19, those of us with chronic illnesses like ME/CFS and scientists researching those illnesses had already been in a kind of trench warfare with public health agencies for decades. Now millions were developing problems that looked just like ME/CFS. All from the same virus. All at the same time. One lifelong advocate, Rivka Solomon, herself an Epstein-Barr virus "long hauler" sick since the 1990s, summed up the situation neatly on a PBS *NewsHour* segment in April 2021: "It is beautiful to see this. It's like the old-timers helping the newbies, but the newbies have much more political clout and are also helping us."

The rarity of the opportunity wasn't lost on Sbrana, who was not quite an old-timer, but not exactly a newbie either.

"We're getting a lot of attention and invitations from federal agencies," Sabra said, "agencies who had previously not treated people with ME well at all…CDC, NIH, etc. All of a sudden I was boots on the ground and leadership within this organization that was getting the red carpet rolled out for them by the NIH, by the CDC, by the World Health Organization. It was like, 'Oh my God, this is the opportunity of a lifetime for a person with ME, knowing what our history has been.' When those groups are rolling out the red carpet for us, obviously we need to take the opportunity, but it is our responsibility to hold that door open and get as many people, advocates from chronic illness communities like dysautonomia, mast cell activation syndrome, whatever, through the door behind us as possible before it is closed."

The Solve ME Initiative, founded in 1987 and the oldest running U.S. patient organization operating in the space, saw the historic opening to reframe the whole political conversation about post-viral disease. They pivoted to campaign for proper research funding into Long Covid, and most importantly, actually help chronically sick people improve. They cheered when Congress included the large $1.15 billion check for research into the long-term effects of Covid infection over four years, which was passed as part of President Biden's massive $1.9 trillion American Rescue Plan stimulus bill.

Solve ME also worked with Republican Rep. Jack Bergman and Democratic Rep. Don Beyer to introduce the COVID-19 Long Haulers Act, a $93 million piece of legislation. This additional bill, if passed, would allocate funding for other health agencies with $30 million for development of patient registries and biobanks via the Patient-Centered Outcomes Research Institute. The proposed legislation sought $33 million for the Agency for Healthcare Research and Quality and Centers for Medicare & Medicaid Services to research and provide recommendations, including improving healthcare access for veterans, low-income communities, the disabled, and elderly communities. The Long Haulers Act also called for $30 million to go to the CDC to help educate Long Covid patients, medical providers, and the public about symptoms, treatments, and conditions related to Long Covid.

The bill's most ardent champion was Emily Taylor, who had been working as the advocacy director for the Solve ME Initiative for five years, starting on her birthday in June 2016. After working in advocacy for a group catering to Black and Latino children with autism, she moved to join Solve ME to help her mother who had been stricken with ME/CFS in 2008, and for whom Taylor was a caregiver. In those five years with the group, she hit a lot of roadblocks in her battle for more research funding, with even a few million more dollars counting as a big success.

"Invisible" illnesses seemed nebulous and hard to define. Only about a fifth of the more than one million Americans with ME/CFS have received an accurate diagnosis, according to the National Academy of Medicine. When people got sick, they often stayed sick long-term. There was no Relay for Life or Walk to End Alzheimer's, and few, if any, fully recovered survivors were able to go out and raise awareness or funding. An interest group couldn't thrive on Capitol Hill if patients couldn't actually get diagnosed in their doctors' offices.

From that vantage point, Taylor saw how scientific research was more successful the more targeted it was. Therefore, the problem of winning funding that might one day cure her mother's multisystem illness was tied to how research funding could be isolated in individual domains or silos. Private foundations and the government gravitated toward specific projects focused on specific organs or specific diseases, but ME/CFS could plausibly be rooted in a range of different specialties. In October 2019, on her last advocacy trip to Washington before the pandemic lockdowns, a congressional staffer asked her if the problem was so big, why was nobody talking about it?

"If all of these people got sick at the same time or in the same place, this would be on the front page of every newspaper in the United States," she told him.

A few months later, future long haulers all started getting sick.

"I wish I wasn't right on that one because I hate that it took so many people getting sick for this to finally be acknowledged," she told me. "I'm glad that it's being acknowledged but it shouldn't have taken this much pain and suffering."

In the years just prior to the pandemic, the NIH had been allocating $15 million annually to study ME/CFS, and now there was a financial influx of nearly a hundred-fold that could truly map vast swaths of essentially unexplored post-viral terrain.

"Suddenly with the $1.15 billion flowing, you see private foundations and government agencies taking a step back because we're starting with a new disease, Long Covid. We're starting to understand it based on past information but it is new data, new experience, new triggers," she said. "I do believe wholeheartedly, with every ounce of my being, that if we solve Long Covid, it will also solve ME."

Taylor co-founded the Long Covid Alliance, which would become a consortium of more than a hundred groups of patients, scientists, and drug developers focused on educating clinicians and policymakers and accelerating research around post-viral illness. The alliance backed Senators Bill Cassidy of Louisiana and Kirsten Gillibrand of New York, who introduced a new bill, the Covid-19 and Pandemic Response Centers of Excellence Act, aiming to create at least ten new Post-Covid Centers of Excellence around the country, hubs that combined clinical care and research. The White House Covid-19 Health Equity Task Force adopted the PLRC recommendations presented by Davis and McCorkell, meeting on June 25, 2021, which called for post-Covid clinics to not require a positive PCR test, which many long haulers didn't have, particularly those with less accessible healthcare.

"I'm really tired," McCorkell said. Though her own Long Covid symptoms had decreased significantly, she kept at the fight alongside her fellow patient researchers, mindful of how she had been thrust into a position to help guide policies that could aid millions of others.

Advocacy burnout is not a new concept, but adding the physical and medical state of many of the Long Covid patients contributes to the weight on their individual and collective shoulders.

Throughout that time, the Body Politic representatives weighed in at each meeting of the American Academy of Physical Medicine and Rehabilitation (AAMP&R) as it gathered evidence from dozens of post-Covid clinics to write consensus recommendations of best practices from Long Covid clinics around the country. More than eighty Long Covid clinics had sprung up in the U.S. during the first year of the pandemic, but each clinic was likely only able to handle between ten and twenty patients in a given week. This way its guidance could inform the organization's more than ten thousand specialists in physical medicine and rehab whether or not they were part of a specific post-Covid clinic or not.

"It's been incredible to see the patient-led team take it to the next level, driving research and being extremely vocal about what questions need to be asked, what research needs to be supported and what's happening at a policy level at the NIH," observed Dr. David Putrino, the Director of Rehabilitation Innovation for the Mt. Sinai healthcare system, and an author of one set of the AAPM&R's guidelines around Long Covid. "We've really enjoyed interacting with the team, co-authoring pieces of work with the team, and having them involved with consensus documents that we're making in the United States, having them on every single call when we decide how we're going to educate physicians about Long Covid."

One major contribution from the patients, he explained, was in clarifying language around post-exertional symptom exacerbation as the most common experience among the vast majority with Long Covid. And they pushed back on psychology-forward language that could hint that the illness was psychogenic, rather than organic in origin.

"It's not that anyone is disagreeing on these points. It's making sure the language is crystal clear and can't be construed that way. We need the patients to be like 'When you say that, this is what we hear,'" Putrino said. "What's important about patient-led collaboratives and making sure their voices are heard is that so few of us as clinicians have walked into a clinician's office and been gaslit. We don't know what that's like. That's the piece of the experience that we don't have."

Chapter 5

A LIFELONG MISSION

I AM A LONG HAULER, of a sort.

It was a different decade and a different infection. But it was the same ensuing chaos, the same devastating fatigue and brain fog, the same lack of understanding from doctors and society. And with the fruitless parade of medical appointments came the same puzzled expressions from physicians, the same nagging existential question of whether some deep subconscious urge within me might somehow be creating symptoms, rather than an actual physical cause.

It was the same questioning of what truth even is.

I intimately know the same symptom constellation as Long Covid. Overwhelming fatigue, unrefreshing sleep, headaches, body aches, brain fog, and strange rashes.

As a high school junior, I saw a series of young flight surgeons at Robins Air Force Base, a sprawling installation on the plains of central Georgia two hours south of Atlanta where the military had stationed my family. Though blood tests came back negative for antibodies to the Epstein-Barr virus, one of the doctors had diagnosed me with mononucleosis. It's a good guess for doctors who see a high schooler presenting with severe fatigue, even if the lab tests don't immediately back it up. Mono can spread via saliva, and since my cross country and soccer teams all shared the same water bottles, I easily could have been exposed to dozens of teammates' germs in a day. For most people, about four weeks of rest is enough to get back into the classroom or onto the playing field. While we know that I was exposed to the virus at some point, as the vast majority of humans are, it's unclear exactly how big a big a role it played in me getting sick.

Prior to falling ill, I had become an Eagle Scout, been elected president of the student council, and was taking several Advanced Placement courses, while also working in a student rocketry team through NASA. Each day at school I also had an hour-long weightlifting class and ran five miles during cross country practice in the afternoon. Several evenings a week I had soccer practice with games on the weekend. Every Friday after school, I hurried to the mailbox to retrieve the week's issue of *Time* magazine. Reading it cover to cover each week, I followed the rise of a young U.S. senator from Illinois named Barack Obama. I fell in love with the art of great writing through its columnists. My goal was to win acceptance into West Point or Princeton on the way toward becoming an Army Ranger, then a writer, and then perhaps one day to run for Congress. I was determined to make a significant contribution to the world.

But when I fell ill, I felt like a mass of inanimate flesh, as though the life force—which usually lit up my body and under-girded its every function and motivation—had simply vanished. There was matter, but there was no energy. I would lie still in a darkened room, because even processing a small amount of light required internal energy that was no longer there. At times, it was the most I could do to raise my head up off my pillow, sitting up in just the slightest way, before resuming the fullest rest position again.

I saw four different primary care doctors along with a neurologist, an infectious disease specialist, an endocrinologist, two rheumatologists, a chiropractor, and an acupuncturist. The countless blood tests never seemed to register an abnormality or known disease. Given only ten minutes, a psychiatrist determined I was depressed and recommended antidepressants. In the parking lot, my dad and I chuckled over the absurdity of the idea, and I crumpled the prescription form in my hand. Antidepressants weren't going to address the underlying condition.

No matter what we tried, I did not improve. The insomnia was impossible to shake, or even to describe.

"I'm too tired to sleep," I told what was probably the second or third young flight surgeon on the Air Force base with whom we'd scheduled an appointment. I thought he'd know what I meant.

"That doesn't make any sense," he replied.

Mono was the first of what would become a long list of misdiagnoses. I pinned a list on our refrigerator with a list of conditions that physicians believed they had successfully ruled out: diabetes, hypoglycemia, heart problems, an active infection, multiple sclerosis, spinal meningitis, brain tumor, cancer.... The list kept growing.

Some of the tests may have been worse than the disease. Strapping electrodes to my head and watching me over a night tossing and turning in a sleep lab didn't yield results showing brainwaves indicating sleep apnea or narcolepsy. The neurologist prescribed Provigil, a stimulant. At the time, it seemed logical: I was always tired, slept too much, and couldn't focus. I took the drug, and immediately felt *alive* again. Though I had missed tryouts, the school's soccer coach had kept a spot open for when I got better. The next day I showed up for a team scrimmage. Within a minute of running after the ball, it was evident something was off, and after a few more, I realized I needed to get off the field before I fully collapsed and needed to be carried off. I slumped in a motionless heap on the sideline, dazed and unable to speak, while the free-wheeling scrimmage carried on just yards away. After what seemed like half an hour, I picked myself up, and slinked off the field undetected. I bawled as I drove home, red-faced and snotty, knowing that I had no chance of getting better in time to play that season. I was mourning losing my opportunity at a starting position on the varsity squad, but in that emotional purge, I was also mourning the loss of a part of myself. It would be years before I would learn that this was called post-exertional malaise, and come to understand why a few minutes on the field had crushed me so severely.

The grief and illness had its own place of suffering, but the groundlessness—which accompanies an illness no one had a template for—is its own brand of torture filled with confusion and hopelessness. Psychologists often refer to something called a "cognitive template." It's a reference point, a way that humans understand our reality and the complex experiences we go through. But when there's no reflection of our experiences in the world, we struggle to make any sense of it at all. Such is the case for chronic unknown illness. It's a no man's land both in medicine and popular culture, where individuals are left to create their own coping mechanisms, emotional and physical support structures, and roads to recovery.

About five months into that bizarre medical odyssey, that same neurologist performed a spinal tap, injecting a needle in the base of my spine, pulling out fluid to be tested for meningitis. I was instructed to lie flat and still for an hour afterwards. It was the first day of March Madness, and I stayed as motionless as I could muster, flipping channels among various NCAA basketball games. Either he screwed up the test, or I fidgeted just enough afterwards to prevent blood from clotting at the base of my spine to close the hole. The resulting spinal leak fluid triggered severe headaches for days after that made it impossible to stand up, but which could be relieved by staying in a supine position.

I couldn't make it to school. Though the county school district was sending teachers to our house to administer tests and tutor me through physics and trigonometry, I still needed to show up for the Georgia High School Graduation Test, which determined whether or not I was worthy of a diploma. That was an issue because spinal fluid leaks cause headaches so severe you can't hold your head up for more than a minute or two before you get nauseated enough to throw up or pass out. I managed to make it to the classroom for the test and laid my head on the desk, squinting sideways at the test booklet, and filling in answer bubbles. I passed.

On repeat appointments to an infectious disease specialist, we racked our brains about every foreign country I'd ever visited, hoping the doctor might be able to link my symptoms to some past infectious outbreak. We'd lived for three years in Okinawa, visited Korea and Hong Kong, had traveled to England twice, and vacationed throughout the Caribbean. But none of the regions had diseases that matched up with my illness, and test results came out clean. One of the visits, as he was screening for sexually transmitted infections, he pointedly asked me if I was sexually active. I told him no. He told both of my parents to leave the exam room. Then he asked me again. My answer was still the same.

As we were leaving the doctor tracked us down in the parking lot, his white coat contrasting the black asphalt and glinting in the Georgia sun, just before we could open the doors of my dad's 4Runner. He asked, "Is it OK if I still test you for HIV?"

Yes, we said. Anything. Anything you can think of.

My subjective list of symptoms—without significant lab results to provide objective confirmation of how I felt—felt like it lacked credibility.

So at each appointment, we followed a calculated strategy designed to build credibility with the doctors. My father, an Air Force colonel and a pilot, often made a point not to change out of his uniform or flight suit when he took me to appointments. Similarly, I often wore a tie, another move calculated to convey the seriousness of our mission. My mother, a registered nurse, kept meticulous records of each appointment, each blood test, each doctor's suggestion of what *might* at least help. She built an exhaustive spreadsheet detailing every avenue we explored, interpreting the cryptic abbreviations in doctors' messily hand-written medical records, and providing her own commentary on whether doctors were making the right decisions or not. Her decades of experience in hospitals and clinics, along with a fierce Mama Bear demeanor, cut through what might have been years' worth of medical bureaucracy in a matter of months, especially when I was often barely well enough to sit up or think clearly for more than twenty minutes on an exam room table.

My HIV test was negative, just like all the others. In that situation, a lingering doubt pulls at you. Maybe there isn't actually anything wrong with you and you've somehow hoodwinked yourself into thinking there is.

One disease kept coming up in all my late-night web searches: chronic fatigue syndrome. But largely because there were no approved treatments, my doctors were reluctant to assign the diagnosis, essentially shirking responsibility for helping me get my life back. Referring us to yet another specialist felt at least slightly productive. After an hour-long head-to-toe examination, my second rheumatologist put her face in her hands. "I believe you. I can tell there is something wrong with you," she said. "I just don't know what it is."

The most formative experience of my life taught me to question the point of the medical profession. As it was failing me, I felt as though there was something faulty about the entire way Western science had gone about the structuring of truth itself, subdividing the human experience into a seemingly endless number of medical specialties. My illness overlapped with a good number of those disciplines but had no natural home in any of them. I could tell many doctors cared, but they were boxed in by a medical bureaucracy that only allowed short appointments, their arsenal populated by pharmaceutical drugs that often did me more harm than good.

Torturous as they were, these experiences were a crucial process of gathering data, building a base of empirical evidence about what did and did not work, and at least providing assurance that I wasn't in immediate danger of dying.

The infectious disease specialist eventually made the diagnosis of chronic fatigue syndrome, handing us a newly printed CDC brochure on the disease and assuring us that the public health agency had made some progress recently. However, that "progress," I found, constituted a CDC public awareness campaign, but explained nothing resembling an actual treatment breakthrough. In a press conference to launch the campaign in November 2006, CDC Director Julie Gerberding said that the agency "considers chronic fatigue syndrome to be a significant public health concern, and we are committed to research that will lead to earlier diagnosis and better treatment of the illness." Official treatment recommendations largely told doctors to send patients home to manage their symptoms as best as they could on their own, that there were no approved drugs, and that the disease could be permanent. That guidance didn't suggest there was any direct path to rejoining the varsity soccer team for my senior year of high school.

With a lifetime of ambitions ahead of me, those lines on the CDC's brochure were like a laceration to the soul. I had to take a full stop in life. In those long periods in which I could do little more than lie in bed with the lights off, I began to develop an outsider's perspective on existence. I learned that the only way to fight my disease was to stop fighting it. Deprived of superficial markers of identity, such as leading my school's cross country team as captain, I had to reconstruct my idea of who I was and how my body worked alone and in the dark. Deprived of my physical strength, I found a new ability to see spiritually. I thought of how astronomers placed the Hubble Space Telescope in orbit around Earth to gain a clearer view of the stars, free of atmospheric debris. Here, too, liberated from the tyranny of the everyday, I gained a broader view of life, through which I could build a new self.

A SOLUTION OF SORTS

In February 2008, I convinced my parents to drive me two hours to the northwestern Atlanta suburb of Marietta to see Dr. Karen Bullington. Medical insurance generally didn't cover her services or treatments, but in more than a year of desperately scouring the Internet, I'd come to believe that her clinic dedicated to Lyme disease, fatigue, and fibromyalgia might be my best shot at regaining a normal life. In most appointments up to that point, I'd had to explain a collection of disparate symptoms to puzzled doctors. This was different. Dr. Bullington would complete my sentences for me if I stumbled, already knowing what I'd planned to say. Such specialists are rare. It's estimated there are only about a dozen full-time experts in the U.S. treating ME/CFS.

One of my parents would drive me to Marietta each week for the IV infusion, which contained about a dozen vitamins and minerals. This functional medical treatment is not approved by the FDA, but since no treatment is greenlit for the disease, patients are left to navigate a gray area of clinical trials, experimental treatments, and alternative therapies. Rather than addressing the root cause of the illness, these therapies often can only attempt to relieve symptoms. Because many patients exhaust dozens of treatments, finding them all ineffective, some settle for a doctor simply willing to listen. Bullington's method was centered around supporting metabolic pathways in the body that were likely broken. It was as though my body were a bucket with holes in it, she said, and the goal was to fill it up faster than energy could drain out the bottom.

I swallowed twenty pills, mostly supplements, each day. I gave myself a vitamin B12 shot once a week and returned to the clinic monthly for the IV infusion. I cannot claim to know of any silver bullet; I do not know a secret that can immediately cure the other twenty million or so people around the world with the condition. All I can say is that it seemed to be working for me. Many simply remain sick for decades, despite trying many of the same things I've tried, plus much, much more.

It was, with constraints, a life.

I was admitted into the University of Georgia's Honors program, joined a fraternity, studied development economics abroad in South Africa, started a political magazine on campus, and interned in Washington, D.C. at *Newsweek*. But I often felt I was the sickest healthy person I knew; or, in some circles, the healthiest sick person. There were still frequent symptom flare-ups that could leave me homebound or bedridden for three or four weeks. I knew little of the invincibility that supposedly marks one's early twenties. Several semesters I teetered on the edge of dropping out of school.

In my last semester of college, I was named a collegiate correspondent for *USA Today*, for which I wrote a weekly story from the perspective of college students. A political junkie, I often wrote about how the 2012 presidential campaign was unfolding on campuses around the country. But in mid-September, an important study by Dr. Ian Lipkin, a renowned microbiologist at Columbia University, had been garnering headlines, disproving a link between chronic fatigue syndrome and a retrovirus called XMRV, or xenotropic murine leukemia-related virus, which was known to cause cancer in rodents. During the past few years, research teams had been racing to try to repeat a 2009 study that had appeared to show a majority of patients had the virus in their blood. However, repeat studies showed the original "breakthrough" study was likely due to a lab contamination mistake and XMRV wasn't ever actually implicated. Had XMRV been confirmed as the true underlying cause, it would have marked a dramatic sea change in how CFS was perceived, diagnosed, and treated. When I caught wind of it a couple weeks later, I chose a big chair in UGA's Miller Learning Center, camped out, and hammered out a more personal *USA Today* column headlined "The real story of chronic fatigue syndrome," laying out my own backstory and why insights from that study mattered. Even though the new research didn't point to a specific cause of the disease, ruling out viruses mattered. Most important of all, I felt, was just the prospect of how media attention to the medical mystery might spur greater interest from scientists to crack CFS in the future. I described the "existential weight of knowing the smartest physicians around had no clue what was wrong with me and could give me nothing to ease my suffering." I recalled how "in those darkest, weakest moments when your body is nothing but dead weight, you learn to see God most clearly. You are reborn."

The response to the story from readers was tremendous; it was the most resonant piece of writing I'd published to that point in my life. I received messages from around the world ushering me into a global patient community I never knew existed. I spent days alone in my apartment with my MacBook poring over emails from people who felt truly *seen* after reading the piece. Some had grievances, explaining how using the name chronic fatigue syndrome belittled the severity of what sufferers experienced as a lifelong neuroimmune disease. And "chronic fatigue" was just one of the numerous symptoms, excluding the flu-like pains, sleep dysfunction, neurological overstimulation, and post-exertional malaise, for instance. The term fails to address the underlying disease process.

I was haunted and inspired by the ways in which readers' stories rhymed with mine. Each followed a similar format. "I was a successful *scientist, lawyer, stockbroker, teacher,*" patients would write, filling in their beloved vocation, affixing a description of their vibrant life running marathons or raising toddlers or racking up stamps on their passports. But for each, a viral infection had changed everything, leaving their bodies permanently dysfunctional. Many had a date, such as February 2, 1992, to which they could point as the moment on which the disease stole their life. Their experiences, often far more torturous than mine, accumulated en masse in our shared consciousness, becoming a form of collective wisdom.

They became my tribe, our fates interwoven, united by a commonality written into our cells.

After graduation, I was finishing up a fellowship researching nuclear nonproliferation for a think tank, while also volunteering for my local congressman's office. My then-girlfriend, Nicole

Castillo, aspired to produce social justice documentaries. She was working two part-time jobs for local TV news stations in central Georgia. We both hungered for something more. After my *USA Today* story, I had been staying in touch with a Canadian woman who hoped to reprint the piece in a self-published book. Over many meandering phone calls, she patiently educated me on the global biomedical and sociopolitical context of ME/CFS research, and why the disease was so misunderstood, all of which she planned to cover in her book.

One night I met Nicole on her break between newscasts during the late shift to take her out for dinner at an Asian stir fry joint. Some combination of arrogance and ignorance led me to believe that we could travel the country filming a feature-length documentary about the disease. I asked her to quit her job and join me in an uncertain journey, not knowing how we would get paid and with no guarantee of success.

She said yes. Immediately.

The course of our lives pivot around a handful of key moments, islands in time with the potential to launch a million future voyages in any direction. For me, that instant, the two of us in that restaurant booth, was one. Had she demurred, I feel, the landscape of my life would be vastly different.

Within a few months we felt rich with about $22,000 via the crowdfunding site Kickstarter, formed a non-profit corporation, and were lugging a trunk full of film equipment out of San Francisco International Airport en route to scheduled interviews throughout the West Coast.

CHAPTER 5

A COMMUNITY'S COLLECTIVE STORY

On our shoestring budget, Nicole had arranged a free bedroom for us to stay in a sorority house on the Stanford campus where one of her friends was managing a pre-college academic summer program. We had scheduled an interview with a professor named Ron Davis for the next day. His daughter Ashley had reached out when she heard we were making a movie, as she had started a non-profit to help her dad raise money to research the disease because her brother was affected by it. Before I fell asleep, I punched "Ron Davis" into Google, to get a sense of who he might be and to jot down some questions to ask him. The Wikipedia entry for him said that he had earned a PhD at Caltech and conducted postdoctoral research at Harvard under Nobel laureate Jim Watson, who, as part of the "Watson and Crick" team, had discovered the structure of DNA. A worthy protégé, Davis became a founder of the field of genomics. He held dozens of patents for building technology that would power the Human Genome Project, mapping every gene in the human body and revolutionizing modern biology. *Whoa.*

"Nicole, come read this!" I called across the dorm room.

If anybody could coordinate scientists to cure the disease, I thought to myself, it might be Davis.

The next morning, Nicole told me that since I clearly couldn't pull off looking like a high school girl and wasn't allowed to be there overnight, I needed to stay in the room out of sight until everyone had departed by 9 a.m. Having woken up and not had a chance to pee, by 8:50 I was dancing back and forth, watching the clock to find out the precise second I was permitted to make a mad dash down the hall to the bathroom. Once we were ready to go, we punched the address for the Stanford Genome Technology Center into the GPS.

A few months later, *The Atlantic* published a story headlined "Who Will Tomorrow's Historians Consider Today's Greatest Inventors?" Davis was one of nine, featured alongside Elon Musk, the founder of Tesla and SpaceX, and Jeff Bezos, who built Amazon.

For Nicole and me, making the film was also a coming-of-age tour of Americana, both majestic and macabre. We hit the road and found our souls. We nearly slept in the rental car with our equipment near Lake Tahoe, Nevada—the site of original CFS illness clusters in the 1980s—before finally finding a hotel room around one in the morning. We were told to quit filming in Grand Central Station (turns out you need a permit for "commercial" shooting on city grounds) while doing establishing shots ahead of interviews with doctors affiliated with Mt. Sinai Hospital. Another night we stayed with a patient outside Boston—who reported that the house was the childhood home of Elizabeth Short, the victim of the infamous Black Dahlia murder—before later that day trudging through knee-deep snow in western Massachusetts for shots with a novelist who had the disease. We bonded with a family in Orange County, California, whose daughter was forced to drop out of college due to the illness. And after a long day of shooting in Fort Lauderdale, Florida, we cracked open beers with a computer scientist who gambled his career to keep researching post-infectious diseases even though funding was often scarce and intermittent.

In New York City, we boarded a train that meandered upstate along the Hudson River, past picturesque little towns on the western bank, en route to interview journalist Hillary Johnson. In the 1980s, she had written a series of stories on the illness for *Rolling Stone* that would receive some of the most reader mail of any article to that point in the magazine's history. She won a book deal and spent much of the next decade reporting and writing her 720-page magnum opus *Osler's Web*. Its title is a reference to Sir William Osler, often considered the father of modern medicine, who championed the priority of listening to patients.

Published in 1996, the book remains by far the most serious journalistic investigation into ME/CFS. It chronicled the lives of doctors during the 1980s across the country who struggled with an onslaught of patients with this mysterious disease. Meanwhile, they contended with internal machinations at the CDC and NIH, as key figures within the agencies treated it as though it is a psychiatric ailment without any real physical cause.

In one particularly startling section, the book details the process in 1987 by which scientists at the CDC and NIH settle, by collaborative process, on the name "chronic fatigue syndrome," instead of other contenders such as "persistent viral syndrome," "chronic mononucleosis-like syndrome," and "myalgic encephalomyelitis," which had been used by British doctors to describe the same symptom phenomena for decades. The CDC's name, chronic fatigue syndrome, which patients nearly universally consider demeaning, unscientific, and vague, also carried with it a set of diagnostic criteria that required patients to test normal on two dozen different lab tests in order to exclude every other disease. It also carried a large dose of stigma. It is a "garbage pail" diagnosis, a dumping ground of sorts for patients who don't seem to fit anywhere else. It's particularly discouraging that even in the 1980s Johnson had interviewed countless scientists and doctors who had substantial data for dozens of different markers of objective abnormalities in their patients across nervous system, immune systems, and endocrine systems. For instance, Dr. Nancy Klimas, then a clinical immunologist at the University of Miami, showed in a 1990 paper that patients had a host of abnormalities, most notably a decreased function of natural killer cells, which fight against tumor cells and cells infected with virus. And Dr.

Anthony Komaroff, of Harvard Medical School, had published a paper in the journal *Annals of Internal Medicine*, looking at 259 chronic fatigue patients from one medical practice, in which he and colleagues found a pattern of problems. "Neurologic symptoms, MRI findings, and lymphocyte phenotyping studies suggest that the patients may have been experiencing a chronic, immunologically mediated inflammatory process of the central nervous system," Komaroff and his team concluded.

Johnson was the first journalist to uncover a pattern in which funds allocated to the CDC's program to research the disease had been systematically siphoned off into other research areas. A 1999 government audit would later show that between the years 1995 and 1998, just 43 percent of the $23 million in the agency's budget for CFS was confirmed as spent for its intended use. Members of Congress had earmarked the funds for research in response to calls from constituents who were disabled by the condition. But when so much of the research that should have occurred was simply shrugged off, expert opinion around ME/CFS would calcify, with many physicians considering the disease an albatross. Many post-viral patients' bodies could be like a crime scene gone cold, and the killer potentially still at large. According to Johnson's reporting, the disease was mostly just dismissed, with those misspent dollars furthering the disease's slippage into the kind of no-man's land that I was plunged into when I fell sick in 2006.

Some eighteen years after her book's release, I asked Johnson how a severe and prevalent disease could slip through the cracks. Was it malice, incompetence...or something else? Her comment to me was as much a lesson in journalism as it was in human nature. There wasn't a conspiracy, but there was a situation in which certain leaders had failed to step up. It's a conspiracy of silence, she said.

With continuous fundraising throughout the production, we eventually earned a total of $150,000 and shot nearly 100 interviews in nine states with scientists from Stanford, Harvard, and Columbia, as well as with journalists who had covered the illness for the *New York Times* and the *Wall Street Journal*. Our company became a 501(c)3 non-profit called the Blue Ribbon Foundation, named after the disease's awareness symbol. We hired an editor who became like a brother to us. We brought on an animator who had worked for Cartoon Network to help bring some of the molecular biology we discussed in the interviews to life. A college friend, in graduate school for music, wrote a score for the film and even assembled a whole choir to record parts of it that would become the soundtrack.

My journalistic journey investigating the disease was the film's narrative through line, but the most enduring images were those of Stanford geneticist Ron Davis and his son Whitney Dafoe, a former photographer, who had become so disabled by ME/CFS that he had lost the ability to speak or to eat solid food. His case had stemmed from a Coxsackie B infection while he was traveling in India. He never fully recovered, and he slowly degraded over time. Entering his early thirties at the time of our visit, he had been bedridden in his room for years, needing his parents, in their sixties and seventies, to care for him.

Ron Davis would come to lead the Open Medicine Foundation's Scientific Advisory Board, attracting several Nobel laureates to join him on a quest to somehow save his son's life, and, in doing so, potentially breathe new life into millions around the globe with the same curse. Both he and his son became, and remain, a symbol of hope for millions. However, to his chagrin, his lab's success in landing massive research grants to map the human genome did not translate to the tens of millions of dollars he felt might be required to radically shift outcomes associated with ME/CFS. Davis sought two NIH grants, totaling $9 million, to seek biomarkers for the disease. He was denied. He chalked it up to a kind of systemic bias within the agency. For the first time in his career, he needed to shift toward private fundraising.

The story of a brilliant scientist's thwarted quest to cure his desperately ill son became the central metaphor for the larger struggle of the patient advocacy movement: hope and innovation were held back by stigma and neglect.

Reflecting on our journey exploring a land of the sick who were hidden just out of view from most of society, we titled our film *Forgotten Plague*. It was an attempt at capturing the scope of the desolation we'd seen. We did our best to seek out inspiring stories of how high-tech scientific advances promised to tease out the root cause of ME/CFS and many similar hard-to-treat diseases, stemming from an infection that never seemed to go away. It was a grassroots project fueled by passion and discovery of the unknown.

It was evident that the problem wasn't so much scientific as it was political. The scientists we interviewed, I felt, were more than capable intellectually to solve it. But, according to a study released as we were filming, less than 30 percent of medical school curricula contain information about ME/CFS. The disease was in the shadows and needed light. But, in science, light doesn't come cheap. And researchers need funds to run their genome sequencing machines, lease supercomputing time, or run randomized control trials. And they need wages to feed their families while pursuing the work. Private foundations sometimes came through with windfalls. In one instance, the Hutchins Family Foundation injected $10 million into ME/CFS research at Columbia University's Center for Infection and Immunity led by Dr. Ian Lipkin. *Discover* magazine called Lipkin "the world's most celebrated virus hunter" following his 1980s research into the spread of HIV in San Francisco and the origins of SARS in China in 2003, as well as for his work as a consultant on the Warner Bros. film *Contagion*. But the only sustainable and large enough source of money was the federal government's National Institutes of Health, and it would likely require pressure from Congress to increase the budget line for ME/CFS research.

Like Davis, Lipkin also stewed when one of his NIH grant applications didn't work out, despite his stature and track record. So patients self-organized a crowdfunding effort called the Microbe Discovery Project with the goal of generating $1 million for Lipkin and fellow researcher Dr. Mady Hornig's plan to investigate how viruses, bacteria, and fungi disrupted or dysregulated the immune response of ME/CFS patients. Lipkin remarked on a conference call that it was as though patients were forced to organize a "bake sale," advocates told me. In 2015, as part of the crowdfunding campaign, Lipkin recorded a video in the Chili ME Challenge. He and Hornig ate spicy peppers on camera in a gambit analogous to the ALS Ice Bucket Challenge, which had gone viral the previous summer. Eventually the NIH came through with a $766,000 grant to complement the $220,000 the patients scraped together.

Science plodded along, and the NIH budget for the disease inched upwards. It wasn't enough to finance the comprehensive agenda needed for a biomarker and a cure, but the scientific base was breaking through bit by bit into the mainstream.

PARALLEL LIVES

Life's purpose can be found, to sum up a concept from Aristotle, where the world's greatest need meets our own greatest skill.

That notion became central to my being as I charted a course in the world after the film.

A high school connection helped me get my foot in the door at CNN's world headquarters in Atlanta. I began with operating teleprompters, miking up on-air guests, and running scripts for anchors across CNN's flagship domestic television network, its international network, and HLN. Starting off in a freelance gig the first year gave me the flexibility to continue leading my documentary team. We finished sound mixing, prepared the digital cinema package, and formatted the film for Amazon Prime and other streaming platforms. I also paced the studios, in between shows, fielding phone calls to organize a fellowship program to educate medical students about ME/CFS and similar neuroimmune diseases.

One day in 2015, sitting in a television control room after finishing a shift working on an international sports show, I joined the first-ever video conference for the board of the #MEAction Network. I'd been invited into the new organization founded by Jennifer Brea, a former Harvard PhD student who became disabled with ME/CFS and went on to direct her own documentary about the disease, called *Unrest*, which won awards at Sundance. Our co-founder, Beth Mazur, had graduated from MIT and ran a website called HealClick where patients with chronic illnesses met to discuss treatments. She had developed ME during the H1N1 flu pandemic in 2009, so was essentially an H1N1 long hauler.

I recast my life. As I started climbing the CNN network ladder, I moved up to clocking in forty hours each week at CNN assisting with 2016 election coverage. I dedicated off time, weekends, and a chunk of my salary to health advocacy projects and speaking at film screenings. I had two lives, running in tandem. Over the next five years, #MEAction would grow into one of the largest grassroots ME advocacy organizations in the world. No matter the success of our online growth, the most vital programs we offered were in our in-person actions and demonstrations held annually in dozens of cities around the world. The events were designed to attract attention from politicians and the media, but for many of us the most profound value came in the solidarity of connecting with patients, families, and allies directly.

On a hot day in Washington, D.C., in May 2016—a day before Donald Trump would officially clinch the GOP presidential nomination—I told my story, speaking through a megaphone, at the inaugural Millions Missing demonstration, in which fellow advocates placed hundreds of empty shoes on the pavement in front of the headquarters for the Department of Health and Human Services. "Millions Missing" refers to the millions of patients worldwide missing from their lives, families, or jobs, as well as the millions of dollars missing from the federal research budget to address the problem. Afterwards, I met with health policy aides for my district's congressman. I also met with a legislative assistant to GOP Senator Bill Cassidy, a physician from Louisiana interested in changing NIH's research funding strategy to prioritize the diseases with the greatest burden to society. #MEAction spearheaded dozens of such meetings, to further our research funding goals, and I would return to Washington, D.C. to educate aides on Capitol Hill again and again.

It's common for advocacy groups representing all kinds of diseases to plan an annual national lobby day, with patients and their families descending on Washington by the hundreds to tell their stories and push their policy priorities. Often wearing the same colorful t-shirts, they meet with their representatives in what I feel is the same moving expression of democratic values that you study in your high school civics textbook. This is the lifeblood of representative democracy, elected officials hearing the concerns of their constituents and using their power to try to make a difference. I spoke to one idealistic Senate aide who relished these meetings as a highlight of her job, hugging and crying with families, promising she would lobby her senator to support their "ask" of increasing research funding or tweaking a policy so that whole swaths of the population might get access to new forms of care.

Medical research funding is one of the few areas in Washington untouched by partisanship. None other than former House Speaker Newt Gingrich had penned a 2015 op-ed in the *New York Times* bearing the headline "Double the NIH budget." He argued that doubling the nation's primary commitment to biomedical research, about $30 billion at the time, was the smartest way to find new treatments for diseases, so the government could take a bite out of the significantly larger $1 trillion it was spending each year grappling with the human costs of those diseases through Medicare and Medicaid.

"As a conservative myself," Gingrich wrote, "I'm often skeptical of government 'investments.' But when it comes to breakthroughs that could cure—not just treat—the most expensive diseases, government is unique. It alone can bring the necessary resources to bear."

If you cure diseases, Gingrich was saying, you cure the spending problem.

Advocates for ME/CFS had been following that same basic line of reasoning for years. Our disease was costing the U.S. economy an estimated $17 to $24 billion in direct medical costs, and lost wages for those disabled by it. By contrast, a similar disease, multiple sclerosis, had only about one-third of the patient population and half the disease burden—measured in years lost to death and disability—compared to ME/CFS. Yet it commanded more than $100 million each year. By this logic, according to one analysis, federal funding levels for ME/CFS ought to have been $203 million annually. However, the NIH budget in 2017 allocated $15 million for researching the disease, some fourteen times less than would be needed to achieve funding parity.

I testified about my experiences before the Georgia House of Representatives' Health and Human Services Committee and helped shepherd a resolution, HR 170, through the full body. It urged the state's public health agencies to commit more resources to helping ME/CFS patients. Similar resolutions carried that year in 2017 in a handful of other states. Each year, the momentum around Millions Missing demonstrations kept snowballing, expanding to more than 100 cities around the world by 2019.

Policymakers were sympathetic, but we bumped up against larger crises—such as the opioid crisis and the specter of rural hospital closures—which ate up brain space, political capital, and open slots in the legislative calendar. Just like everyone else, policymakers only had twenty-four hours in the day, and they were preoccupied by whichever fires burned the brightest.

In response, many advocates chose to personalize the message, telling legislators that this same horror could happen to you or your family. Though the message aspired to a sense of urgency, it still risked making the disease seem like a more abstract, lower-level concern compared with other systemic health issues that commanded a greater share of the public's attention.

I was just one of thousands who played a role, in a mass effort in which each person contributed their own particular skills or perspectives or personal style.

I earned a main stage speaking slot at the Stanford Medicine X conference, an annual gathering that celebrated emerging technology in medicine. Measured by social media impressions, it billed itself as the most discussed academic medical conference in the world. Importantly, it was one of a growing number of venues that highlighted the voices of patients in guiding scientific research. Working on health advocacy had originally served to build an audience for *Forgotten Plague*. This role later scratched my itch to be involved in politics, and throughout had fulfilled me with constant messages of gratitude from severely ill patients in need of a voice. But the Med X speech invited an opportunity for greater intimacy. I dug deeper to reflect on my truest reasons for so many hours of work that offered no immediate personal payoff. Though I had negotiated a fragile truce with the disease, my deeper fear was that it would eventually fully disable me, just as it had done for so many of my friends.

Projected on the huge screens behind me were images of Ron Davis and his wife Janet Dafoe hunched over, looking after their son Whitney, who was gaunt and scruffy. Then we flashed to a young man named Jamison Hill, a former bodybuilder who developed ME/CFS, and who had lost the ability to speak or to eat solid food. There were no obvious differences between Jamison, Whitney, and me. Why had I become able-bodied, virtually recovered? They had not.

At the edge of my every thought was the inescapable notion that the disease could be like a ticking time bomb, conspiring, one way or another, to detonate my dreams as well.

"I want to teach my son to build a fire under the starry sky. I want to teach my daughter to dance the salsa," I told the audience at Stanford. "I fear that I would join the thousands of parents who miss piano recitals because they're disabled by a disease the medical establishment doesn't really recognize. I'm twenty-seven now. And I don't want it to be this way when I'm forty-seven."

A PERSONAL LENS

In his classic book *Man's Search for Meaning*, psychiatrist and Holocaust survivor Viktor Frankl begins with the premise that all suffering, on its face, is devoid of purpose or meaning. But figuring out a way to assign our suffering some purpose, he argues, is one of the most powerful ways of trying to heal from it. It struck me that our experience with profound pain is as valuable to future success as any school, credential, job, or award on our resume. Climbing out of a hole—grappling with an incurable disease, recovering from the loss of child—matters as much as, if not far more than, any worldly accomplishment, such that we continue persisting in what is often a daily test of finesse and endurance, of grace and grit.

From many of my interactions with the ill, it's clear that a livelihood lost to a chronic condition is often a collection of untapped experiential wisdom and resilience. Many have no choice but to live within uncertainty and shame and brave them head-on. Like most internal bullies, they don't survive well when confronted. It's really as though suffering itself belongs on one's resume.

Ought we to consider that enduring a life-altering disease or the soul-shattering death of a loved one could be life experiences as useful as a degree from Yale or a job developing software for Google?

Frankl writes: "There are situations in which one is cut off from the opportunity to do one's work or to enjoy one's life; but what can never be ruled out is the unavoidability of suffering. In accepting this challenge to suffer bravely, life has a meaning up to the last moment, and it retains this meaning literally to the end. In other words, life's meaning is an unconditional one, for it even includes the potential meaning of unavoidable suffering."

Over the decade between falling sick and stepping into a role as a national advocate, I was often sustained by a remarkable piece of writing by the twentieth-century Austrian poet Rainer Maria Rilke laying out how to live your way into becoming a true writer. The excerpt, from Rilke's semi-autobiographical novel *The Notebooks of Malte Laurids Brigge*, reads, "For the sake of a single poem, you must see many cities, many people and Things, you must understand animals, must feel how birds fly, and know the gesture which small flowers make when they open in the morning." Rilke lays out a litany of experiences, both epic and mundane, spanning the variety of human existence.

The piece continues on to "childhood illnesses that began so strangely with so many profound and difficult transformations, to days in quiet restrained rooms and to mornings by the sea, to the sea itself, to seas, to nights of travel that rushed along high overhead and went flying with all the stars—and it is still not enough to think of all that."

Eventually it reaches a kind of mysticism I found mysterious as a college sophomore, but which has come to feel familiar as I've grown: only when these experiences "have changed into our very blood, into glance and gesture, and are nameless, no longer to be distinguished from ourselves," Rilke writes, "only then can it happen that in some very rare hour the first word of a poem arises in their midst and goes forth from them."

At age sixteen, I had aspired to attend West Point to earn a commission as an Army officer and eventually become a Ranger, a direction not so different from Rilke's, who had left military school around that age due to an illness. I built and led the Blue Ribbon Foundation, a task that required studying as much about molecular biology as it did the IRS tax code. I had grown close with men and women living with ME/CFS who connected us with scientists, donated their savings, and organized film screenings. But what had begun as giddy youthful idealism and an all-too-ready willingness to absorb the triumph and tragedy of the world had turned far darker. More than half a dozen patients and advocates that I worked closely with had actually taken their own lives, choosing death after decades of unshakeable suffering instead of living with it for decades more. That's in keeping with studies showing that these patients are at a six times greater risk of suicide than the general population. Many of those memories, too painful to process or to recall from the mind's depths, became like a blankness on the consciousness, biology's way of preserving an organism that's grappled too closely with oblivion. Buddhist nun Pema Chödrön, who herself grappled with chronic illness, captured the notion beautifully, writing, "Only to the extent that we expose ourselves over and over again to annihilation can that which is indestructible in us be found."

On stronger days, I knew the grief might just be the cost of idealism, another signpost on a road toward collective redemption, provided there were those who could keep bearing the message.

Those experiences, both remembered and forgotten, were now transmuted for me into blood and glance and gesture. During the pandemic, they were a lens for gazing into Long Covid, a new version of an older disease.

Chapter 6

WE PREDICTED THIS

FOR THE CHRONIC ILLNESS COMMUNITY and those attuned to the history of outbreaks, the rise of Long Covid was utterly predictable. The initial idea that survivors would get sick for a couple weeks and recover was a fantasy. The novel coronavirus was of course novel, but even the most similar previous virus, SARS, had left long-term sickness in its wake. A host of other pathogens causing other pandemics had also shown a similar capacity.

One of the people best able to grapple with that prophetic fact was Leonard Jason, a professor of psychology at DePaul University, who had been studying the aftereffects of infections for three decades. After falling ill with ME/CFS in the 1990s, Jason spent much of his career studying the condition, developing an understanding of the various case definitions and the epidemiology of the illness. As the pandemic hit the U.S., Jason and his team were crunching data on a four-year study of mononucleosis in college students, designed to yield insights into which people would recover slowly, and which might not recover at all, developing chronic post-viral syndromes.

They studied about 4,500 college students, watching who would be infected with the Epstein-Barr virus, develop mononucleosis, and then suffer long-term illness afterwards. They found that 238 of the students in their research cohort were diagnosed with mono, which usually doesn't last more than six weeks. However, Jason found that of those who developed mono, fifty-five of them, or 23 percent, went on to meet the definition for ME/CFS six months later, and 8 percent developed cases of severe ME/CFS.

Behind that data are dozens of stories of students whose trajectories unexpectedly bent toward disability and oblivion, who disappeared from their normal social relationships and academic goals. From just a small sampling of Chicago students over a few years, you can't help but try to imagine the personal costs behind a failure to recover from viral infection. The students in the study could represent dozens of PhD applications gone blank or missed roles in symphonies, not unlike the Body Politic's Alison Sbrana in Colorado a few years earlier.

If you just knew what to look for, and how to design a prospective study to capture it, the data and the humanity of post-viral illness are hiding in plain sight.

"If you look at all the pandemics from the Spanish flu on down, a certain number of people never get better," Jason told me. "At least ten percent six months later seem to still be having symptoms. With Covid-19 I think the rates could be very much higher."

He and colleagues summed up perspectives from a century of post-infectious syndromes with a research article published in June 2020 entitled "Post-viral fatigue and COVID-19: Lessons from past pandemics."

This historical data helps give us context based on epidemiological precedent. The medical community ought to have been better prepared to handle the emergence of Long Covid. For instance, one study Jason highlighted found that of 1,000 patients who survived the 1918 flu, some 200 did not fully recover, reporting symptoms that worsened with physical exertion. The data showed that forty of them, or 4 percent, remained severely ill.

The degree to which people experienced long-term effects after a major infection varied, but they showed up in outbreak after outbreak. At their onset, each virus or bacterium could present in its own way. However, the long-term effects tended to look very similar regardless of the original pathogen.

For instance, a 2006 study conducted in Australia followed patients infected with Epstein-Barr, Ross River virus, and Q fever at regular intervals over the course of twelve months. At the end of six months, 11 percent of them met the criteria to be diagnosed with chronic fatigue syndrome, suffering disabling fatigue, musculoskeletal pain, neurocognitive difficulties, and mood disturbances.

A study in Houston, Texas published in 2008 followed patients who had come down with severe West Nile virus infections. It found that eight years after onset, more than 40 percent of patients with the mosquito-borne disease had symptoms including fatigue, muscle weakness, difficulty walking, and memory problems.

Similarly, some 28 percent of those recovering from Ebola virus experienced debilitating levels of fatigue in the first year after infection as well.

The exact on-ramp into the post-viral syndrome could differ, but they all looked similar afterwards. "There are some that are more and some that are less," Jason told me. "And we're clearly trying to figure out what the rates are with Long Covid. But it's in the ballpark."

The closest evidence of long-term consequences was a study published in 2009 that looked at people in Hong Kong who contracted the original SARS virus. It showed that 40 percent of patients reported chronic fatigue still ongoing four years after their original diagnosis, with 27 percent qualifying for a clinical diagnosis of ME/CFS. More than a quarter of those with the first SARS virus were irrevocably changed by the infection. While the mind can easily conjure up an image of frailty, disability, and gravitas at the mention of ALS or multiple sclerosis, there isn't a similar collective mental schema for ME/CFS. The horror can't be easily portrayed in a memorable visual form.

It's impossible to fully channel the level of inner human tragedy lurking behind even a single one of those statistics. The "fatigue" captured in these studies is not the common everyday fatigue of sleepiness after lunch, burnout from a chronically too-full schedule, or flagging energy after going too long without a meal. It can be a profound failing of the body to produce energy. Period. A growing scientific consensus believe there's likely some kind of a wrench in the machinery of the mitochondria, the organelle that acts as a power plant generating energy for each individual cell. It's a deficit in the fundamental molecules whose tiny metabolic processes animate a spirit of life into otherwise inorganic matter. It's a feeling of being a slender waving reed knocked over by even the gentlest passing breeze.

Likewise, the oft-cited "brain fog" masks its own failing in the English language; it is a colloquialism nowhere near up to the task of expressing how whole mental faculties disappear, how memories recede, how words cease to exist, how even the meaning of a single street sign becomes like an indecipherable ancient text. How tiny decisions cause you to go blank. Brain fog is the blinding inability to produce coherent thought.

We ought to have a single iconic image for that unique devastation. For me, the moment early in the pandemic—of reading about the long-term effects from the first SARS virus—conjured

Edvard Munch's 1893 painting *The Scream*. You've surely seen the painting or at least seen it referenced in pop culture. It's a wavy Expressionist rendering of a human figure. Its palms are held up to a face, with eyes wide open, and mouth agape in an existential shriek as though of an "infinite scream passing through nature," the painter later wrote. The figure—situated on a public walkway, yet alone in its despair—sits in the foreground of an ominous blood-red sky. Its face is widened at the top, more like a 1950s alien than a natural human visage.

The scientific literature is clear that post-viral fatigue syndromes follow epidemics. But the quiet desperation they unleash in individual lives struggles to penetrate the public consciousness. The international conversation is centered on quantifiable metrics of death counts and hospitalizations. Covid skepticism can flourish when infection and recovery are seen as an all-or-nothing binary, rather than a game of Russian roulette with the risk of lifelong disability. Many cases fall into shades of grey.

A "CHIEF MAD SCIENTIST" TAKES ON LONG COVID

In short, the problem of post-viral disease cried out for innovation, for aggressive problem solvers willing to run into the fire to tackle tough challenges that everyone else had abandoned saying it wasn't their problem. Thinkers who weren't worried about being rule followers. At Mt. Sinai Hospital's rehab innovation lab at the outset of New York's outbreak, Dr. David Putrino was in a unique position to take leadership in the space, blazing a trail from the trenches of the pandemic toward the cellular makeup of a forgotten illness.

His job was to quickly translate strong science into quality clinical care, combining a startup founder's "fail early, fail fast" drive with the sophistication of a medical professor. Putrino earned a PhD in computational neuroscience, with stints at MIT and Harvard. For his work using cutting-edge technology to improve the lives of people with disabilities, the government of Australia named him Global Australian of the Year in 2019. He could see how the process of rigorous, deliberative clinical trials was necessary to make progress in medicine, but they could also seem at odds with to the bold, driven thinking required to accomplish a task quickly.

"In any organization, you have mission-oriented people and you have compliance-oriented people," he told me. The tension between the two poles is perhaps most pronounced in a hospital, where moving fast and breaking things will likely get a doctor sued. "During the pandemic, it was all mission-oriented. Just get out of the way, come up with solutions to help people navigate the crisis."

Free to be himself, Putrino could harness a lifetime of experiences that highlighted the importance of listening closely to patients and using those values to drive the direction of treating Long Covid. As the usual institutional red tape fell, his roots as a neuroscientist and a physical therapist set him up to pioneer the first stab at solutions.

RETHINKING REHAB

During his postdoc, Putrino worked on a project designing a robotic arm with a brain-computer interface, a challenge that illustrated the importance of empathy and human-centered design in achieving effective results.

"I was the only clinician. Everyone else was an engineer," he said. "Everyone was viewing these brain-computer inter-face technologies as an engineering problem that needed to be solved, not as a clinical problem with a patient at the forefront. I saw the really challenging limitations of forgetting that person that you're developing technology for."

During the early years of his career, Putrino also volunteered as the "Chief Mad Scientist" of Not Impossible Labs, a group that crowdsources accessible technological solutions for high-impact humanitarian problems. In one Not Impossible project, Putrino helped a boy named Daniel from a war-torn village in South Sudan's Nuba mountains. Daniel needed both of his arms ampu-tated following a bomb blast and was undergoing an existential crisis about his future. They 3D-printed a prosthetic arm for him and set up a lab where the villagers could continue printing more prosthetics for others. That type of direct problem solving was critical to helping disrupt a field. Even if it wasn't the ultimate holistic solution, it was a spark of innovation showing what was possible, inspiring others to come in and build further.

"It was about the ability to just show up, work the problem, and see that solution be implemented. That was really powerful and really meaningful," he said. "I like research and I like aca-demia but sometimes it's nice to go out and solve a problem in a weekend. You see the solution, and get to work."

In directing Mt. Sinai's rehab innovation efforts, Putrino oversaw three different centers. One was Performance360, which worked with the athletes from the U.S. Olympic team, the NBA, and the NFL. There was one center focused on care for kids. And another focused on new technologies for people with neurologi-cal disorders, which came to include Long Covid.

"I like to have a very broad scope working with high-per-formance athletes all the way through to individuals with ALS, who are completely locked in, and across the entire lifespan from newborns to older adults," he said.

Balancing sports performance and neurocognitive rehab made it possible to learn from people everywhere on the spectrum of human ability. Some ALS patients, for instance, with bodies degenerating toward paralysis, could summon immense cognitive resilience and focus during the most seemingly minute of tasks. They scored off the charts in measures for psychometric traits that clinicians wanted the NBA players and baseball players to have. Likewise, insights from the high-performance athletes could directly apply to neurocognitive rehab patients. NBA players benefited from working with a coaching team every day to individualize their training, making it engaging and exciting. They knew exactly what exercise they were doing and why it would enhance their performance at game time. On the other hand, stroke survivors don't always receive the same level of direct clinical attention. They were slow to improve when told to perform a thousand repetitions of a movement without an explanation as to why, and without the investment in them of a professional sports club hungry for a championship. Most therapists "don't even watch them do the movement because it's boring to watch and we kind of just wander away. And we expect them to just recover with that standard of coaching and training," Putrino said. "So one of the things we do in our clinic is we bring that level of emotional salience and engagement into our rehab process, and our outcomes really speak to it. We have a lot of people who come to us to recover from a stroke and they gain a lot of function in a short period of time. The science would say it's because of the approach we take."

They experimented with virtual reality, immersive rooms, and video games that add the virtue of turning the thousand reps into something exploratory and engaging and fun. Those experiences in innovation guided his team as they engineered outside-the-box ways to collaborate with patients in the first studies of Long Covid.

Prior to the pandemic, Putrino's lab had built a remote patient monitoring mobile app called Precision Recovery, designed for stroke patients to track their blood pressure after they've left the hospital. About a quarter of those who have strokes can wind up re-hospitalized with a second stroke. The best way to prevent that is by monitoring blood pressure. But that's not always done in conventional care, where patients get discharged and might follow up with primary care every few months. So, Putrino and his team onboarded several hundred people post-stroke into their app, where on a daily basis they could collect blood pressure and information about the person's general well-being.

Then the pandemic struck. By the end of March 2020, the Mt. Sinai Hospital hit a point of building tents in Central Park to reckon with all the overflow from the emergency department. The biggest struggle many clinicians reported was in figuring out what to do when a patient showed up with a definite case of Covid but wasn't sick enough to be admitted to the hospital. They needed to be closely watched.

"I still remember at that time, in my lab we had a whiteboard up, and we were just counting down the number of available beds in the health system," Putrino explained. "So it was like, we don't have enough beds to take everyone in who's symptomatic, but you also don't want to say the advice was go home and come back if you're sicker."

That prompted them to redesign the Precision Recovery app to focus on identifying someone with Covid-19 at risk of respiratory failure, with questions around the intensity of the patients' fevers or blueness of the extremities. Pulse oximetry was the most obvious metric to measure, giving objective data on whether the virus was causing someone's blood oxygen levels to plummet. They started buying up every pulse oximeter they could find in the city, but they ran up against a shortage as customers all over the country ransacked store shelves. In the early months of the pandemic, the shoe company Zappos announced that its customer service team would help with any customer service task, *anything*, even chatting about your feelings if you needed it. Putrino tweeted at the company asking for help sourcing pulse oximeters. Someone from Zappos directly messaged him back, found him 1,000 pulse oximeters, and delivered them to the hospital in the midst of the shortage.

"We were either same-day shipping pulse oximeters or we had a team of interns and myself and we were just getting in a car and driving around the city and hand-delivering them to people who were on-boarded into the app," he said.

They launched the new program in a matter of forty-eight hours, at times making personal house calls to drop off monitoring devices to patients. Walking up to houses of Covid patients in $25 million mansions in Greenwich, Connecticut, or low-income housing in the Bronx, it was painfully clear to him how Covid-19 cut across all of society. Their process enabled people to monitor themselves from the beginning, logging symptoms and oximetry results into the app interface. For anyone who showed signs of deterioration, the app included a basic algorithm to signal to the core clinicians monitoring them that they might need medical attention.

The majority of users tracked their symptoms and vitals for a few weeks, felt better, and were sent on their way. However, about 10 to 15 percent of the people they were tracking with the app stayed on past five or six weeks and were no longer reporting acute Covid symptoms. Instead, they complained of dizziness, headaches, and crashes after exercising. They couldn't remember names and had to search for words while speaking that wouldn't come to them.

"We would have this daily huddle where we would talk about the difficult cases. Should we send this person to the hospital? Or, what should we do with this person?" Putrino said. These cases were nowhere near recovery but also not severe enough for hospitalization; rather, they were somewhere in between. Many patients didn't feel confident and well enough to quit the monitoring app. By the end of April, the team had the first inkling that they were dealing with a post-viral illness.

"I feel really fortunate that because of the diversity of what I do, we had this team that was meeting about this who came from all walks of life," Putrino said. "We had cardiologists, we had psychiatrists, we had a pulmonary physiologist, we had a bunch of physical therapists, a strength and conditioning coach and a nutritionist. We had two clinicians who had Long Covid themselves."

Well before the pandemic, Putrino's innovation lab embraced a core guiding principle of community co-design, a "nothing about us without us" mentality. In building a new technology or treatment program, they didn't design anything for a disease without people living with the condition or disability in the room telling them what they needed to improve their lives.

"Otherwise, we usually fail," he said.

With newly sick Long Covid sufferers enlisted within their own ranks, they didn't have to go far to get patient input. As they were building surveys or brainstorming ways of measuring signs of the illness, members of the group piped in saying, "If you do that to me, I'm going to be useless for two days."

They connected with a group of hundreds of clinicians in the UK who had Long Covid, and by late May they started meeting with the Body Politic crew.

CO-DESIGNING AN INITIAL
TREATMENT PROGRAM

"I think the Body Politic quickly passed us in terms of just the diversity and number of different symptoms that they were seeing because of the data they had from people just openly sharing their data on a forum like that—versus having to wait for [Institutional Review Board] approval and ethics approval," he said. Putrino joined the Slack group and wrote back and forth directly with the members. *Are you seeing this symptom? Yep. Are you seeing that symptom? Yep.* As clinicians, their goal was to learn from the patient collaborative, to wrap their minds around the scope of the illness and discern how similar it was to post-infectious syndromes seen in the past.

Mt. Sinai pulled together its Center for Post-COVID Care in mid-May 2020 to try to address what were emerging as the major issues: the fatigue, cognitive impairment, and post-exertional symptom exacerbation. Clearly there were a lot of symptoms driven by autonomic nervous system dysfunction, and one key first step would be finding ways to quiet the system down.

Just before the pandemic, Putrino had been chatting with a certified breathwork coach, Josh Duntz. A former Naval Special Ops veteran, Duntz used to disarm bombs for a living. Duntz noted to Putrino that after a particularly taxing flights in which fighter pilots pull a lot of G's—enduring gravitational forces many times the norm during hard turns and acrobatic loops—they often develop symptoms that sounded a lot like Long Covid. The fighter pilots have hypocapnia, or low carbon dioxide levels in the blood. During a mission, pilots' lives depend on knowing how to control or prevent these symptoms. Duntz had noticed the difference in his own life, with breathwork helping power him through longer endurance runs with a slower heart rate.

And sure enough, once Putrino's team started testing long haulers for carbon dioxide, they saw the same problem, and published a study showing that almost three-quarters of people with Long Covid have hypocapnia. Duntz started training long haulers in a kind of breathwork that helped increase and retain their CO_2 levels. In a basic version of the exercise, you inhale through the nose for a count of four, and then exhale through the mouth, counting to six. The program enables patients to control their own heart rate. It helps calm the body's fight-or-flight response, and it could help modulate the immune system.

The Mt. Sinai team paired the breath work with very gentle autonomic rehab techniques, which eased many of the symptoms. Once they could demonstrate that they were at least effective as a basic measure against Long Covid, they trained more than 700 physical therapists around the country on the same techniques. These protocols do not eliminate the problem, not by a longshot. They're akin to slapping on a Band-Aid as a temporary fix before diving more deeply into the pathophysiology of the disease. It's possible to move the dial and achieve about 20 to 30 percent in improvement after three or four months of careful and gentle rehab, breathwork, and nutrition management, Putrino told me. At that point, long haulers were still in the position of managing a chronic condition. With easy, effective treatments hard to come by, a new life as a chronically ill patient meant always walking on eggshells, following guidelines around pacing oneself in daily life, and prioritizing accomplishing only the most basic or essential task so as to avoid another crash and symptom relapse.

"We are by no means saying this is the cure, but we are saying that people who follow these rehab protocols tend to experience a reduction in their symptoms," he said.

The complexity of the diseases defies the medical profession's usual reliance on an algorithm, a set concrete protocol for treating disease. For Long Covid, there was no algorithm. Instead, clinicians had to be patient-centric, focusing on a particular person's direct condition and experience and teaching them how to avoid their symptom triggers, such as new food sensitivities or intense reactions to heat or cold.

Chapter 7

COVID
FOR CHRISTMAS

ON CHRISTMAS EVE MORNING 2020, I awoke to a cryptic voice-mail from the director of a commercial testing lab. I had stopped in for a Covid-19 nasal swab test a day earlier. The lab director asked me to call him back. When I got hold of him, he was brief: "It's positive."

I'm not sure where I was exposed. I'd spent ten months wearing a mask, generally avoiding gatherings, and using hand sanitizer. When people ask me how I contracted Covid-19, sometimes I just shrug and say, "By living in the United States." During the winter wave of 2020, the virus was everywhere.

Home for the holidays, I isolated in my parents' expansive basement in Woodstock, Georgia, about thirty miles north of downtown Atlanta. We kept our interactions brief, masked, and distanced, usually just for a meal delivery three times a day. On Christmas Day, our family opened presents over FaceTime, and I squinted at an iPad screen as my niece and nephews opened picture books I'd wrapped for them. Since I was quarantined, that night I drove over to my brother Jason's house to deliver some more stocking stuffers, where I was told unceremoniously to just leave them on the porch.

Friends volunteered medical advice, a pulse oximeter, vitamins, a Disney Plus password, and an HDMI cord, which I used to hook my laptop up to a TV I drug out of the storeroom. Patients and experts I'd interviewed over the previous year reached out to share treatment tips. My energy didn't rebound quickly. I was in bed early on New Year's Eve and managed to respond to a couple celebratory post-midnight texts before I drifted off.

I tweeted that I had tested positive for Covid. Among the flood of condolences, there was Hannah Davis. She told me she couldn't do much, but perhaps I might like to join the Body Politic group on Slack? She sent me an invitation.

Just after New Year's, I logged into the group, where more than 9,000 people with Long Covid had gathered to share their experiences. I dashed off a post in the introductions channel explaining that I had tested positive on December 24th, and that while many of the initial flu-like symptoms had subsided in a couple days, I'd been left with persistent and consistent fatigue. The symptoms shut everything down for me by about 7:30 or 8:00 each evening. I would lie very still until about 11 p.m. before needing another eleven or twelve hours of sleep to get moving again.

Within a few minutes, I received a response from a man whose profile indicated that he was a guitarist, a Christian, an IT specialist, and one of the leading "data nerds" on the platform. He explained that I could look at charts detailing the responses from nearly 4,000 Body Politic members, each of whom had filled out a 257-question survey. Through that data, I could glean more insights into the experiences of others with the same complaints. The survey responses wouldn't make my symptoms go away, of course, but at least a sense of solidarity would be reassuring.

As a reporter, I had worked with the Body Politic numerous times over the first nine months of the pandemic. That usually meant filing a request via their online form, explaining the story I was writing, what types of patients I might like to speak to, and my deadline for publication. A member of the Body Politic's media team would post my request in the Slack group, and patients would email me if they wanted to be interviewed. Membership in the group was only for patients, by invitation only. There's a sanctity to those kinds of conversations among communities of shared sufferers, and it shouldn't be violated. Not by companies marketing a product. Not by conspiracy theorists gawking at the conversation or heckling their discussions. Not by journalists selling a story. But now I was inseparable from the story. I was living it.

Over Christmas, I had read the pre-print version of their upcoming medical journal article based on that same survey, which members of Body Politic's patient-led research team had analyzed in conjunction with university researchers.

I never had trouble breathing, never was hospitalized, and never lost my sense of taste or smell. At least in my case, the initial mild cold was just a minor set of jabs while Covid prepared a vicious uppercut with its other fist.

KEEPING THE LIGHT ON

As the light fever, cough, chills, and body aches from the first few days of Covid gave way to a different kind of illness, it felt like a deep, malicious, alien force had entered into me. It reminded me of a moment from middle school when our biology class was roaming our campus casting about for bugs and other animals we could later dissect. A group of us had wandered off from the class to a cow pasture encircled by an electric fence next to the school. Curious, each of us took turns grabbing hold of the wire, until the deep otherworldly punch of electricity pummeled us, forcing us back. Two weeks into the virus, the force of Covid was eerily reminiscent of that direct voltage.

I was grateful to be in Atlanta, near my family and doctor. Although none of us had experienced Covid, my parents had practice dealing with the same type of symptoms, when I had first gotten sick as a teenager. "This is basically a replay of when you were a junior in high school," my dad said. If asked what I wanted for dinner, the most I could muster was a blank stare. Most mornings, I couldn't walk up the stairs from the basement, and might text my mom or dad asking if they could bring me a smoothie. *Brain fog* felt like a demon wraith had grabbed hold of my mind and sent painful shockwaves throughout my nervous system. In its grip, it crushes critical thinking, problem solving, and language processing skills.

Eight months earlier, I had been accepted into the Harvard Kennedy School for a master's degree in public policy. Prior to the pandemic, my visits to the campus had felt like walking into a cathedral of learning, and I longed to interrogate the many heads of state who jetted in and out of campus on a constant basis, influencing the next generation of world leaders learning there. I had thought the program would open up new vistas of journalistic possibility and hoped the education in policymaking would bolster my ability to build advocacy movements, something we had been working to do with #MEAction. I wanted to spur innovative new approaches to research and drug development, to affect breakthroughs to help my suffering friends. But as the pandemic had gripped the world, I had asked Harvard for a deferral. I suspected that if I contracted Covid-19 while living near campus in Cambridge, Massachusetts, I would be alone in an unfamiliar city as the virus exploited my already compromised immune system. If I were to get sick, I wanted it to be in Atlanta, a fifteen-minute drive from a doctor I trusted with my life and where I could tap into my decades-long support system if the disease were to turn life-threatening.

Beyond that, one of my CNN editors, who was also a Kennedy School alum, explained to me that the most meaningful period of her career as a reporter had been in New York in the weeks and months after airliners had struck the World Trade Center towers. She advised me to stay at CNN, as we shifted to working from home. There would be time to sit in classrooms later, especially if the courses in 2020 would only be held over Zoom. For now, the unfolding weeks, months, and years would reshape the globe for a generation. I was in a position to help tell that story, particularly through personal narratives.

Words from the talk I had delivered at a Stanford Medicine X conference three-and-a-half years earlier echoed in my mind. Speaking about my deeper personal reasons for advocating on behalf of the sick, I had suggested that although I appeared healthy to many people—most of the time—I worried my illness was a ticking time bomb inside me, ready to consume the idealized life I longed for. "I fear that I would join the thousands of parents who miss piano recitals because they're disabled by a disease the medical establishment doesn't really recognize," I had said at the time. In the speech, I'd highlighted new biomarkers for the illness, and called for dramatic new research initiatives to help others. Now was the time when I worried that time bomb might detonate.

I had cobbled together treatments and coping mechanisms over the past decade, braving flare-ups on a roughly annual basis that left me mostly in bed for three or four weeks. I was supposed to be the inspiring one. For many, my life was what the rare "recovery" looked like.

However, lying on a futon in my parents' basement, too weak to walk upstairs for my own food, it was hard to escape the dark suspicion that Covid-19 had exposed my recovery from ME/CFS for the house of straw it really was. I'd been lucky enough to improvise a life—working full-time, traveling, playing some sports—that looked successful on Instagram, but left out selfies of the too-many nights coming home from work collapsing onto my bed in pain, lying there for hours until it was time to sleep. Now, the coronavirus tempest had shattered even that illusion of strength, just as a hurricane throws roofs and walls of houses across a storm-ravaged coast.

I remembered my friend Cindy Shepler, who had given up a high-powered career at Cigna at age thirty-five due to ME/CFS, fibromyalgia, Hashimoto's thyroiditis, and several other autoimmune diseases. Her handful of painful overlapping complex illnesses seemed to play off of one another, not unlike what many would later experience with Long Covid.

I'd met her in her sixties while working on an advocacy project, and we had formed an unusual and deep friendship. She'd poured her enthusiasm into me, becoming my strongest cheerleader, living vicariously through my travels in Europe and celebrating every first date or big story I published. But her diseases had become too much to bear. Accompanied by her husband and with his support, she traveled to Switzerland for a death with dignity, receiving a lethal injection in lieu of more years of continued pain. Granting her last wish by writing what would become my most personal story for CNN, I sipped coffee by the Chattahoochee River in Atlanta transcribing quotes from her final conversation with me just hours before her death, while hospital workers were falling sick in Wuhan, China. If there was one thesis to her life and her mission in advocacy, it was that all immune disorders were interrelated.

Now, a year later and unable to count the number of weeks I'd been unable to work, I worried that Covid was dragging my body one step closer to Cindy's fate. But I still felt buoyed by her love, knowing that in some way, the pandemic might be unveiling truths about human biology she had intuited all along.

And then there was my friend Imraan Sumar, who never graduated from college, used a wheelchair, and who needed in-home caregivers. It all obscured the potential of his brilliantly curious scholarly mind. He seemed to me well-versed in everything from ancient Islamic mystics to the latest debate in parliament. I imagined him as a religion professor, dazzling students with his grace and humor, if the disease hadn't hit him so hard. ME/CFS had dashed the dreams of many I'd come to consider dear friends. I worried that perhaps Long Covid was coming around to destroy what ME/CFS hadn't already taken from me.

Time was slowly losing its meaning, each day a constant return of the same. Every week I had to tell my editors I'd need another week to recover, knowing another week would most likely pass and my state would remain unaltered. On the mornings when I woke up capable of getting out of bed, I had to summon strength to overcome the dread of wondering if I could make it to the next room before a knee-bending pang of pain or nausea or fatigue might strike.

From my Covid reporting before I got sick, however, I knew that millions around the world were in the same situation, struggling with symptoms well past the commonly cited two weeks of illness. Yet those same symptoms, which sapped my energy, cognitive function, and even ability to look at a screen, made it nearly impossible to do deep, substantive research into how to relieve them. Extracting any meaning from the latest scientific journals—a usual standby for a science writer—was hopeless. I tried to read news articles and postings in online support groups, but nearly everything I could find would only note that severe long-term aftereffects were common in Covid, and scientists didn't yet know why. Most patients on support forums seemed to be fumbling in the dark too. My brain fog meant that my mind would go blank halfway through an article, my language processing ability absent after just a few paragraphs. But the headlines told me enough: "Long haulers sick for 10 months with no cure."

Each night my parents flipped the TV on to watch the *PBS NewsHour*. I had become agitated and confused by most sounds and just the movement in the video being broadcast was disturbing to me. If I was in the living room, I had to retreat downstairs to my sanctuary of stillness in the basement, cloistered from the noise. Meditation, a habit that had receded from my life years before, became one of the few ways of relieving symptoms, or at least sorting through the despair so that I could see the biological signs for what they were.

In the absolute stillness, I read, ploddingly, *The Universal Christ*, a book by Franciscan priest Richard Rohr, who argued that God resides in all things. I tried to imagine the divine as the whole extended network of family, friends, colleagues, doctors, and nurses all playing their roles in an elaborately choreographed production meant to make me well.

Many nights, I was devoid of energy and scarcely able to speak a meaningful sentence. My sixty-eight-year-old mother massaged my neck, my back, my limbs. As she kneaded my muscles, I felt as though she was somehow squeezing another half-hour's worth of energy and mental clarity to propel my ragged body just a little further. "I can't believe how good this feels," I would tell her.

I imagined that this was what it was to be held in the hands of God.

PROVING AN ILLNESS

I burned through a year's worth of sick days by the second week of January.

As the illness showed no sign of abating, I had to file for short-term disability insurance coverage, which could cover my paychecks while I desperately fought for my health so that I could return to the purposeful work of telling the stories of the pandemic. I'd filed this before during ME/CFS flare-ups in which I'd needed to receive more IV treatments and recuperate for weeks at a time in order to feel myself again, strong enough to endure the stimulation and pressure of a twenty-four-seven global newsroom.

I got a call from a cheerful insurance claims specialist I'll call Tricia. She worked for the Hartford, the insurance company responsible for handling my short-term disability claim. She chided me like an old friend, because earlier in the pandemic, the clinic supplying the infusions I needed each month had temporarily closed and I'd become too sick to work. Tricia had covered my claim. Although jousting with a giant insurance corporation is many people's idea of hell (including mine), she had somehow made it a joy. She made quick work approving my previous claim. In turn, I had set a goal that I'd be healthy from then on. I vowed to never need her help again.

"You broke your promise," Tricia joked. "But I'm happy to help."

But when I needed to see multiple doctors and manage their process of filling out complex bureaucratic forms, getting a positive result proved much harder. Each time when I picked up the phone, the nurse assigned to my case bombarded me with questions about the date and outcome of my latest doctor's appointments. That level of scrutiny is of course likely helpful in ferreting out whether someone might just be using the short-term disability system to underwrite an extended vacation. But it was invasive and hostile, as though they were doubting if I was actually sick, like every other Long Covid patient not being believed. In my frail state, I had to ask her to slow down, repeat her questions, and explain the definitions of basic terms they used. With a mind that only had a couple hours of good concentration time each day, accumulating the documentation to prove I was still ill hampered my fragile recovery. Every conversation hinged on whether my family doctor had cleared me for my "return to work" date. It made me feel as though the only use for my body— to the insurer, to society at large, to capitalism itself—was to be back on the clock working whether I was ready or not. I was campaigning, however feebly, for the proper time to convalesce. And it felt like I was fighting against the grain of the "work to eat" philosophy underpinning the American way of life.

Each week came and went with little to report in the way of symptom improvement. Getting the bureaucratic paperwork filed properly meant that my two doctors needed to sign off on a specific diagnosis, prescribe a defined course of treatment, and give an estimate for when my brain and body could carry me through another workday of writing and reporting about the pandemic. But the aftereffects of Covid didn't follow a set schedule. One doctor would pick a return-to-work date a couple weeks away just to complete a form. Then, at my next appointment, the other doctor cast it out a little farther, seeing that I needed the breathing room. That, in turn, set off a new flurry of calls from the insurer asking me to fax or email the latest records.

In America, short-term disability policies are policies provided by either your employer or a private company that can last from a few weeks up to twelve months, while long-term disability policies are similar in function but differ in their duration. Both short-term and long-term disability services are distinct from government assistance programs like Social Security Disability Insurance and Supplemental Security Income, where factors such as length in Social Security covered employment and income and asset status come into play. Short-term policy benefits are not guaranteed to all workers in America and vary by employment status, policy, salary, disease, and many more factors. According to the Bureau of Labor Statistics, only 40 percent of workers are offered short term disability by their employer. More shockingly, among the lowest 10 percent of earners, only 10 percent are covered by short-term disability, and 5 percent by long-term disability. Among the highest 10 percent wage group, 64 percent and 66 percent are covered by short-term disability and long-term disability, respectively. Persons with low socioeconomic status are at a higher risk of serious complications from Covid-19 and are less likely to have employer-provided disability insurance. These populations are extremely vulnerable to poor physical and financial outcomes due to a long list of compounding barriers.

Thankfully, in the end, my claim was approved, meaning I was entitled to keep the paychecks I'd continued to receive while I was out. A denial would have meant paying the company back for the months of salary I drew while recovering. I had to return to work, so I started with only half days for the first two weeks. I worked slowly, wearing blue-light reduction glasses—looking at anything was hard, particularly the cold glare of the screen. I played calming Himalayan chants, dropped Nuun electrolyte tablets into my Nalgene water bottle to aid in my hydration, and took breaks to meditate and pool my strength.

Covid had kept me out of work for about seven weeks, from just after Christmas through Valentine's Day. With the two-week period to wade back in, I was back at a normal schedule by the end of February. Even though I was back to working full-time, the symptoms continued to relapse throughout the whole next year. I logged in from home each day for my scheduled shift usually reporting on the pandemic. And I kept wading through test results or treatments with my doctors to find new solutions to the symptoms, testing some new idea about each month.

As violating as the process felt, I'm among the lucky ones who have access to fully paid short-term disability at all, along with protections to return to the same job. I also had two positive PCR tests, proving I really did have Covid. Many long haulers— particularly those who got sick early in the pandemic when tests were in short supply—had to forge into the jungle of medical bureaucracy without even that basic evidence, making their story seem as though it might not hold together. I was also fortunate to stay with my parents while sick, an arrangement that would have been made dramatically harder if I were raising kids or living far from home. And my symptoms, while bleak, weren't nearly as horrifying or diverse as those of many people I've spoken with.

That said, the uncertainty around the symptoms, particularly the cognitive ones, brought its own form of terror. I made my living dwelling in the written word, so knowing how quickly I could lose my dexterous vocabulary was ominous. I became acutely aware of how much energy was involved in even the simplest act, in reclaiming the sorts of mental gymnastics that are second nature to any working journalist.

Getting my abilities back meant first mustering the simple act of writing something, anything. Then came writing with clarity. Next was writing something *complicated* with clarity. From there, I'd have to plot some path toward scaling the imposing mountain of attempting to write something complicated, with clarity, and *on deadline*. Then might come the final step essential to the modern role, of doing all of the above while at the mercy of Slack notifications and incoming email across multiple monitors, each necessary interlude annihilating the slightest pure thought I could steal from the virus.

Put another way, working my way up through that newfound hierarchy of neurological stimuli might start with trying to listen to a soothing podcast, then working up to a news podcast, then the big step toward watching a TV with sound on. After that, I'd have to see how long I could endure the sensory assault of managing all that while somebody else was in the same room with me. At some distant point in the unimaginable future, I might be able to watch TV with the sound on, while others were buzzing and clinking away in the kitchen. In short, the most basic form of social gathering was a pipe dream.

It made me—this is as best as I can describe it—feel like I had the flu. I imagined the remnants of the virus as settled at the bottom of a still lake. But minimal exertion, like even a pebble dropped in the water, stirred up the sediment. My mind and body would again be overcome with muddiness, which drifted out to cloud everything.

AWFUL GRACE

Through a decade and a half of these ups and downs, I've always been comforted by the words of the Greek playwright Aeschylus: "Even in our sleep, pain which cannot forget falls drop by drop upon the heart, until, in our despair, comes wisdom by the awful grace of God."

Each time, I'm reminded of what an *awful grace* suffering can be, that it doesn't have to be wasted time. Sickness can deepen our empathy and appreciation for the plight of others. If my own illness and writing could serve some larger role in the unfolding betterment of humanity, then surely there is a sturdy worth in it. Rather than fighting against it, I could build my existence to harness it, voicing the struggles of those who've been born or forced into lives they didn't imagine. Lived experience was one of the foremost catalysts for large scale policy change. And I heard a similar language in many of the stories I chose to focus on in my writing: a single mom scrubbing toilets for minimum wage, or an activist with a felony record marching on the streets for justice.

That seemed to follow from Frankl's argument in *Man's Search for Meaning*, about how the human yearning to tap into a sense of life purpose is the motivator for our flourishing and for reckoning with trauma. If holding steadfast to purpose in a concentration camp could bolster one's chances of survival, then it could pave a solution to life's myriad lesser challenges as well.

Frankl quotes University of Georgia psychology professor Edith Weisskopf-Joelson as writing that this approach "may help counteract certain unhealthy trends in the present-day culture of the United States, where the incurable sufferer is given very little opportunity to be proud of his suffering and to consider it ennobling rather than degrading." As a result, she writes, "he is not only unhappy, but also ashamed of being unhappy."

A similar stigma snakes into the consciousness of those living with a physical disease. Many of us are not only physically sick, but are also *ashamed* of being sick, bearing the burden of asking for exceptions to rules, accommodations to protocols, in order to compensate for not being able to do what a "whole" person can. Psychologically, shame is one of the more difficult emotions for us to process, as it tightly tugs at our deep sense of worth, adequacy, and even morality. In many facets of our life, shame is a brutal corrector that reminds us when our actions fail to meet our values, and consequently we perceive our social relationships might be at risk. It's not a surface emotion, but one we feel deeply tied to our character.

At first glance, its relationship between shame and illness seems tangential. One reason we experience shame surrounding physical illness, survival, and fitness is an evolutionary one akin to other emotions like disgust. People with illness might experience physical changes that lead to judgment from others and unchecked reactions such as disgust. Healthy friends and family might question what we did to cause this illness and why we haven't taken the correct steps to solve it on a timetable they deem appropriate. We unconsciously or consciously question our own character.

Even our non-sick allies might probe the question of shame itself: Why would someone feel ashamed for something they cannot control? But the fallacy of control is at the heart of a more complex paradigm around shame consisting of deeper questions. One question that permeates is: who is to blame for prolonged illness? And furthermore, as blame is closely tied to shame, who holds the fault in these arenas: the patient or the inadequacies of modern medicine? Notably, these questions illuminate our dogged fixation to decipher causation, many times at the expense of the patient. Historically, people with diseases have been subject to religious scrutiny and suspicion, as divine judgment satisfied the thirst for causation in the place of a scientific explanation.

Inevitably, people with disease begin to question their own value and internalize other people's insecurities, reactions, confusion, uneasiness, and ignorance, and it trickles into the fabric of one's own self-image. In Susan Sontag's famous collection of essays *Illness as Metaphor*, she explores the cultural phenomenon of the "blame the victim" mentality and its internal ramifications as it relates to tuberculosis, AIDS, and cancer. Tuberculosis was known as a passionate disease, where people's internal character traits were seen to progress or heal the disease depending on the trait presentation. Sontag addresses these connections to personality and their correlating metaphors as she writes, "with the modern diseases (once TB, now cancer), the romantic idea that the disease expresses the character is invariably extended to assert that the character causes the disease—because it has not expressed itself. Passion moves inward, striking and blighting the deepest cellular recesses."

Today, the debate as to whether personality and disease are connected is a messy and complex area of study. Do people have "cancer-prone personalities"? Or, more likely, are there immune differences and genetic predispositions at play within individuals that account for both personality and cancer risk, over neither of which we have full control? Either way, sadly, many people suffer the consequences of social isolation as they strive to maintain their sense of worth by avoiding the judgment of others, and thus the accompanying shame. And while we may counter our deepest insecurities of being broken, worthless, weak, or burdensome by reminding ourselves that we are loved, even our most convincing mindful coping strategies cannot always compete with the harmful systemic projections within our culture. No doubt feelings of shame are compounded in patients with complex and poorly understood diseases where medical doubt is present and the existence of disease itself is questioned. It's no surprise, then, that shame is a poison bubbling at the surface of patients with chronic complex illness, as the explicit message being handed down by persons in perceived authority is: *I don't believe you have it, but if you do, you did this to yourself.*

Chapter 8

UNRAVELING
THE MYSTERY

THE FIVE PRIMARY WOMEN IN the Patient-Led Research
Collaborative had their own sets of expertise, in public policy
or user design or computer programming. But Athena Akrami
was unique. She was the only one of those early connected Long
Covid patient researchers who had a PhD and was actively running a neurology lab. She had used her position as a systems neuroscientist at University College London's Sainsbury Wellcome
Centre to sponsor the patient team's symptom survey research
as they shepherded their paper through peer review toward
publication.

As a student in Iran, Akrami had earned her undergraduate
degree from Tehran Polytechnic studying biomedical engineering, but she grew disillusioned with the idea of building objects,
when the humans around her seemed so riveting.

"I was really fascinated by human behavior; specifically
growing up in Iran, there are so many different people with different ideologies," she said. "It's so many characteristics around
you. You just wonder, how can the same brain give rise to one

way of thinking over the other? These really polarized ideologies, where do they come from?"

She had studied for her PhD in Italy, and then spent a long postdoc in the U.S. at Princeton University before settling in as an assistant professor in London. Her research focused on how animals move around an environment and learn meaningful structures "without anybody teaching them," she said. Perhaps the most dynamic example is a baby learning human language, starting with a blank slate, and learning the structure and meaning of basic words by her eighth month of life. "So the final goal of my lab is to understand how we do that. What is the computation that happens at the brain level of this human child, and what are the properties of the neural networks, of the brain structures that make this computation possible?"

In March 2020, however, Covid gave her a new application for computational neuroscience. She and her husband Ryan Low both got sick.

By her fourth week of illness, Akrami had diminished to the point of being unable to stand up or walk, experiencing unexplained shaking, pins and needles numbness in her hands, and a high sustained fever. So, she called an ambulance. Akrami felt what could be driving the symptoms could be a cytokine storm, surges in a type of signaling molecule in the immune system. Cytokines alert other cells to an infection and bring specialized immune cells to help eradicate the invader. Akrami and her father-in-law, retired physician Dr. Russell Low, had been sending studies about cytokine storms back and forth to each other. Early science began to indicate cytokine storms were driving many severe Covid-19 cases, where the body in a sense would go to war with itself, sometimes resulting in death. Akrami showed the articles to the physicians treating her for her Covid symptoms, which deviated from what scientists had originally understood the virus could cause.

"I was with one of the doctors, and was like, 'Have you ever heard of cytokine storms? Do you know about this type of inflammatory response?' And he didn't know about that, but he was very eager to learn." A second doctor, however, shot down the neuroscience professor's effort to illustrate the science of her symptoms. He told her it was just stress.

For the first nine months, even walking for five minutes had been enough to put her body into a post-exertional crash. By January 2021, she found she could walk around for about half an hour each day without crashing, and she could tolerate going to work in her lab once or twice a week. In June 2021, her neurologist finally told her she had small fiber neuropathy, with sharp pain attacks that begin in the feet or hands. She had high levels of various cytokines, including TNF-alpha, which is associated with the body's response in inflammatory bowel disease.

"As long as I don't do exercise, I'm OK. But exercise can induce [post-exertional malaise]. Before that I used to be able to do like three days a week," she said. "Now, nothing."

Along with her husband and father-in-law, she wrote a preprint paper offering a set of hypotheses to explain how the huge range of 203 symptoms seen in the Body Politic group—from neuropathic pain to vision problems to brain fog—could be potentially explained by elevated cytokines generated by an abnormal immune response. The body's central nervous system could be affected either by the novel coronavirus directly, or by an indirect immune response. From there, the chronic low-grade inflammation could disrupt brain cells called microglia, causing them to release central cytokines, which produce neuroinflammation. The primary symptoms experienced by the majority with Long Covid—intermittent fatigue, brain fog, and post-exertional malaise—were likely all related to the elevated cytokines. Finally, the symptoms of Long Covid, they argued, closely mirrored those of ME/CFS, so developing the best possible map of persistent inflammation in Long Covid would simultaneously work as a blueprint of the gateway to ME/CFS.

EVADING THE USUAL TRICKS

Dr. Noah Greenspan, a pulmonary rehab therapist in New York City, found that the respiratory virus was leaving long-term illness, but the symptoms weren't directly pulmonary in nature.

An eccentric clinician with colorful tattoos adorning both his arms, he developed a deep passion for his patients, an intellectual fascination with their illness, and a willingness to do whatever he could to improve their lives at a mass scale. His nonprofit, the Pulmonary Wellness Foundation, ran a virtual long hauler support group on Zoom every Sunday night that fostered intimate conversations among people who were braving the disease without much help from family, or co-workers. Those profound stories prompted Greenspan to produce a documentary film, debuting on the film festival circuit in fall 2021, rooted in the experiences of members for whom the meetings had become a lifeline.

"Covid long haulers come in every shape, every size, every texture, every color, every consistency," he said. And their recoveries were unpredictable. Of the hundreds of patients he'd worked with, some had recovered readily, others improved at a snail's pace, and plenty of them were getting worse over time.

Long Covid challenged his abilities in ways that little else had throughout a career in which he had prided himself on being a kind of precision sniper tackling the toughest cases referred to him. Before, he might encounter a case every three years that really stumped him. Now he was stumped on a regular basis. Every person was like a knotted ball of yarn, and pulling any individual string out from it was an achievement. Or, put another way, it was as though any particular long hauler's case was a time bomb. Cutting one wire might disarm the device; cutting another might trigger a cataclysmic explosion. Even when he tried his best tricks, they didn't always work. The chest pain and shortness of breath so many people experienced wasn't caused by obvious problems in the heart and lungs. The dysfunction in each person's autonomic nervous system expressed itself differently with each person, producing their own particular flavor from the sprawling menu of options by which the body could unravel.

A pig, so to speak, would oink. A cow would moo. Covid might provoke your system to "bark" with headaches or gastrointestinal issues or dizziness.

And though he was confident in the good work he and his team were doing, there was little they could do to scale up the deep painstaking work of sorting through each case individually. No single treatment could help the majority of them. Because there was such tremendous variability, there was no set formula for how to treat every patient.

"For me, that's the most interesting and exciting part of it as a clinician, because it's like you're given this super puzzle and you're having to figure it out," he said. "We've seen every combination of symptoms that either helped, hurt, or were unaffected by various treatments." Any type of overexertion, physical or otherwise, carried the risk of generating post-exertional malaise, triggering devastating setbacks. So, working within patients' fragile energy parameters was key. You throw a little pebble in a lake, wait for a ripple effect, let it calm down again, and then decide if it is safe to drop another pebble in.

KNOWING WHERE TO LOOK

Michael VanElzakker is a neuroscientist with Massachusetts General Hospital, Harvard, and Tufts University. The idea that viruses could hide out in reservoirs in the body and cause disease had tugged at him throughout his career. In the late 2000s, he was working on his master's degree in neuroscience at the University of Colorado at Boulder around the same time as Facebook was gaining popularity. VanElzakker reconnected with an old high school friend, whom he'd remembered as bright and driven. She told him that she had dropped out from early acceptance to law school after coming down with chickenpox. A year later, she couldn't walk up the stairs. Doctors were telling her she had chronic fatigue syndrome, and some didn't believe it was real. "I *know* this person. She had goals and a plan, and for her to stop that, to say she was playing the sick role is just nonsensical," he said. "It's absurd."

At the same time, VanElzakker was learning about the how the very feeling of being sick was essentially a nervous system response, and he knew scientists down the hall and up the stairs who were working out the neuroendocrine circuitry of how bodies create sickness behavior—such as a fever or chills—in response to an infection.

"I was fueled a little bit by just being mad about it," he said, the injustice of his friend's situation serving as fodder to ply his craft. It was common knowledge that the varicella-zoster virus, which causes chickenpox in the young, can hide out in the body for life, triggering painful shingles rashes decades later. Herpesviruses in general are known for their ability to persist. He also knew that the body's sickness response is guided by the vagus nerve, a cranial nerve that permeates the whole body and trunk organs. Vagus, which comes from the Latin for "wandering," is the root for words such as vagrant and vagabond and describes a cranial nerve with wide-ranging connective potential to nerve centers, like an interstate highway. A virus infecting the nerve was like holding a candle up to a smoke detector: a tiny flame could trip the sensor and cause sprinklers to douse a whole floor of a building, even though the fire was tiny. What if VanElzakker's friend's law school dreams had been thwarted by a virus lodging itself somewhere in her vagus nerve, causing a permanent sickness? Could it have left her body in a state of ongoing alert over what should have been a non-issue? There was evidence in rats that concept held weight. He stopped one of his professors, a decorated neuroscientist, in the hall to pitch the idea.

"She said, 'Oh my God. All it took was for someone to put it together,'" VanElzakker recalled. "And those words have fueled me for years."

In 2013, he published his vagus nerve infection hypothesis and immediately attracted the attention of some of the brightest minds in the field, and he started getting calls from donors asking how they could support his lab, or fund a research assistant for him, moves that would amount to a huge leap up the chain of command for a third-year grad student. "I was like, my [principal investigator] would kill me if I have an assistant and she does not," he said.

Eventually he finished his PhD, and a wealthy donor covered his postdoctoral research to better understand ME/CFS through brain scans, but getting the funding for an entire staff and research program proved difficult. During presentations, VanElzakker explained his approach with a cartoon showing a man looking for his car keys under a lamp post, even though he says he actually dropped them somewhere else. So why does he keep looking for the keys under the streetlight? Because that's "where the light is," he says. Just because you can see doesn't mean there's something worth seeing.

There was a similar level of futility in running studies looking for viruses in blood when the pathogen was likely tucked away in some hidden nook or cranny. "You can't just do blood tests over and over again. You're simply going to miss stuff. That's not how the body works," VanElzakker said.

When the pandemic hit and SARS-CoV-2 triggered long-term symptoms in significant percentages of patients, he and microbiologist Amy Proal authored a massive review of the scientific literature, surveying emerging studies charting various pathways by which the virus could persist in tissues, dysregulate the immune system, alter the microbiome, and reactivate dormant viruses. They compared them with research on pathogens such as Lyme and Ebola that were known to seed longer syndromes.

The smattering of evidence collected around the world showed there could be any number of drivers for Long Covid in a particular person, and a quest to discover a single unifying cause for all of it was likely to come up short. One set of variables, for instance, were likely at play in heart palpitations. Another underlying reason would likely explain parosmia, in which someone's sense of smell could be distorted, making a steak dinner come off like rotten meat or flowers smell like garbage. No single person was a truly clean scientific experiment, and the nuances of individual bodies could produce too many different outcomes to count.

"Humans are just filled with all kinds of [microbial] stuff. We're these little Serengetis walking around," VanElzakker said. "Most of us have it reasonably under control." A vicious virus tipping that homeostasis out of whack ought to invite researchers down the path of investigating the basis for inflammation.

His and Proal's overview led him to believe that tamping down a seemingly overactive immune system could cause harm in some cases, particularly if the immune system was actually fighting a real invader, just wrestling with it outside the proverbial street-light under which we're currently capable of seeing.

"When things are termed 'post-viral' that generally bothers me," he said. There may not be any *post* at all.

At the time, the general scientific consensus was that the virus could not cross the blood-brain barrier and directly infect the brain. But that could have been because there hadn't yet been enough high quality studies into the question, to repeatedly prove it. Studies had gone as far as showing, however, that SARS-CoV-2 could infect cells in the central nervous system, and that RNA or proteins from the virus were present in the brainstem during autopsies in both animals and humans, just as occurred with the first SARS-CoV virus. Proving that SARS-CoV-2 could directly infect the brain, if it could, was a more challenging pros-pect. He was intrigued by one German study, which hadn't gar-nered many headlines, that did report finding the virus' RNA in the brainstem.

Overall, though, there was an important question to answer of how SARS-CoV-2 could *affect* the brain and nervous system, or how much of the brain injury occurred from the virus being able to cross the blood-brain barrier and *infect* the brain? All kinds of things can affect cognition and the brain, but broadly speaking, the answer comes back to how inflammation affects the brain. According to VanElzakker, there are three possible routes. First, there's the humoral route via the blood, in which mediators for inflammation can enter the brain through open-ings in the blood-brain barrier, but that's uncommon. Next, there's a cellular route, in which immune cells get dragged across the central nervous system. And then there's the neural route, through the vagus nerve, in which the nerve's chemoreceptors around the body detect local indicators for inflammation and then send alerts up to the brain.

VACCINE HELPS SOME

After a year of the pandemic, all hope of a return to normal rested on rolling out vaccines, thereby spreading immunity in waves across the population. On December 11, 2020, the FDA authorized the Pfizer vaccine for use in the U.S. after results showed that it was 95 percent effective against preventing both mild and severe infection. Moderna's vaccine trials achieved similar success.

Few expected vaccines might have a therapeutic benefit for long haul symptoms, not least of all Geralyn Lucas, an author, breast cancer survivor, and mother of two in New York City. The virus spread within her family in March 2020 when the first wave of infection struck the city. Her symptoms were alarming and required medical attention. When she and her daughter arrived at the hospital, they were greeted by blinking construction signs outside the complex directing drivers not to leave their car or roll down their windows.

"It was just completely bizarre. It was surrealistic," she said.

She hadn't coughed once, but her blood oxygen level was dangerously low at eighty-six when she entered the ER. She was diagnosed with double pneumonia and admitted. Her son received his positive test result as she was being wheeled into the Covid ward, where she stayed more than a week.

"I remember doctors talking to me over microphones, like these disembodied voices. I just thought about my daughter in the parking lot who couldn't be there with me and had to wait in there for hours to find out what was going on." She spoke to her family through a screen, and hospital workers wouldn't come into her room. After she was discharged, she felt long haul symptoms for months. She had a hard time catching her breath, exercising was difficult, she kept coughing up fluid, and awful diarrhea caused her to lose a lot of weight. "My body would do this really weird 'shake' thing. I had tremors, like *shakes*, and buzzing. I couldn't get my body to calm down." She was also easily startled, waking up in the middle of the night shaking and screaming.

A year later, Lucas, still suffering her unusual and unrelenting Covid symptoms and concerned about her immune system being compromised by chemotherapy earlier in life, was terrified to get vaccinated.

"I was so sick. I couldn't find any information about who had long haul or who got vaccinated, so it was kind of a leap of faith," she said.

But she was more afraid of getting Covid again than the vaccine. She had so normalized the awful feelings of diarrhea and shaking that after the first few days of normal side effects, she hardly noticed the subtle feelings of uplift as Long Covid receded. The weight she'd lost returned, she could finally exercise again, and she just felt *normal*. The feeling seemed permanent, like she was back to her usual self. But six months later, the fevers, shakes, and diarrhea returned, as though maybe her symptom relapse coordinated with what studies had shown about waning immunity from the vaccine. In early October 2021, given her immunocompromised status, she was eligible for a vaccine booster shot, and she felt her symptoms lift again.

It left her to wonder how much longer the cycle of symptoms and remission, vaccine and immunity, despair and hope, might keep repeating, her own life a microcosm of the larger unfolding of ignorance, knowledge, and continuing discovery at the heart of science and human life.

Stories like Lucas' are not uncommon. Throughout late winter and early spring of 2021, waves of long haulers reported feeling partially or totally recovered after getting the shot. As with other aspects of Long Covid, patient groups organically generated some of the earliest signs, buzzing with the emerging stories, many months ahead of formal researchers in identifying and cataloging what might be a promising new therapy. As anecdotal stories permeated patient groups and social media, recovered long haulers became a fixture of TV news shows and media stories for weeks.

Several informal patient surveys showed that about a third of long haulers may have found at least some relief, driving scientists to strike out in pursuit of the question. A preprint study by researchers from the University of Paris found that 16.6 percent of long haulers who received a vaccine experienced a complete remission, compared with 7.5 percent of unvaccinated long haulers. This means that inoculation effectively doubled the likelihood of recovery. Well short of a universal long haul panacea, vaccines did, however, have their place as part of the medicine cabinet.

Vaccines are usually designed to prevent diseases, but here was a case where an immunization, administered after someone had gotten sick, seemed to act to as a remedy for at least some patients. It's tricky to say exactly how or why the vaccine could do this, but understanding the underlying physiology of it carried the tantalizing prospect of being a way to unravel the mystery of what caused Long Covid in the first place. Could the novel coronavirus still be active in some hidden reservoir in some people's bodies, driving symptoms? Or, even if the virus itself was gone, could fragments or remnants in the form of stray genes or proteins still be at large, tricking the body into an unnecessary set of sickness behaviors? Perhaps vaccine recoveries would add credence to the theory that Long Covid was the result of auto-immunity, with the immune system remaining in a state of per-manent excitation following the infection, unable to calm itself down again. A vaccine, in this case, might resolve symptoms by teaching the immune system to modulate itself. Vaccines could be clearing out the SARS-CoV-2 viral reservoir or changing the body's autoimmune lymphocytes. Some people even reported Long Covid symptom improvement from a regular flu shot, which could suggest a number of vaccines might have positive immune system effects for persistent symptoms.

Regardless, the vaccine question illuminated the hunt for Long Covid's cause, treatment, and cure along the trend lines of viral reservoir, viral fragments, persistent inflammation, and autoimmunity.

"It could be that a subset of patients only have one of these, or others have a combination of three of these," said Akiko Iwasaki, a professor of immunobiology at Yale University. "Or maybe all of them have some of it. I don't know what kind of breakdown it's going to be."

Iwasaki amassed an enormous following on Twitter during the pandemic, fueled by her belief that educating the public about how viruses and the immune system work was a vital part of a robust pandemic response. She regularly tweeted out answers to basic immunology and virology questions posed by readers online, breaking down the issues into clear, digestible bites. That close back-and-forth discussion translating science for everyday people helped her hatch one of the most promising research projects to get inside the question of why the coronavi-rus was generating so many millions of long haulers. She could read those signs and symptoms emerging from our body politic and synchronize a scientific agenda around them.

"It all started with me looking at the Twitter feeds to see what patients were reporting at the time," Iwasaki told me. "A key drive comes from the patients, what they tell me, how they're suffering from the disease, and what's happening to their loved ones. The emails—unfortunately I don't even have time to respond to all of them—but I read them, and it's devastating what's going on."

To Iwasaki, the most notable patient survey on social media came from the UK-based LongCovidSOS. It looked into long haulers' responses to three different vaccines, with a slim majority reporting at least some improvement after vaccination, about one-fifth saying they felt worse, and the rest remaining the same. It was informal citizen science, to be sure, but the trove of data was of immense value for designing a more robust investigation to discern which immune markers in the blood might be driving recovery or a further descent into illness. Iwasaki referenced the survey "all the time," she said.

Her research group's north star was a belief that patients ought to be equal partners in co-designing scientific studies. The Patient-Led Research Collaborative contributed to the design of the researchers' surveys, along with members of Survivor Corps, a Facebook community that has amassed nearly 200,000 Covid survivors. In this way, the design intimately reflected the full range of patient-reported symptoms and how they relapsed and remitted through the seemingly endless course of disease. And, of course, the patient communities directly recruited participants into the study.

"Patients know best what the disease is," Iwasaki said. "Doctors are just recipients of that information. They know exactly what's going on. They may not know what's causing it, but they know how it feels and what their symptoms are, and whether it comes and goes."

People whose careers have cratered or whose children struggle to attend school can't have answers fast enough. But the timelines of human suffering and careful diligent science are divergent, at least in the agonizing unfolding present.

"It's such an urgent need, but I don't want to do half-baked science where we lead to the wrong conclusions," she said. "So I think I'd rather take my time to do the study appropriately with the right number of participants."

For their ongoing Yale COVID Recovery Study, Iwasaki and her team signed up long haulers prior to receiving their first vaccine. The patients filled out validated symptom surveys and gave their blood and saliva for a baseline analysis. Researchers would draw blood and saliva twice more, at six weeks following vaccination, and then again twelve weeks out from the shot. From there, they would be able to compare how changes in patients' immune responses might result in changes in their symptoms.

Beyond just Covid long haulers, the animating question behind the study suggested avenues into understanding larger questions in human biology, and how other types of diseases might have a similar pathogenesis. Only in recent years have we begun to map a more accurate understanding of brain diseases, which points toward possible infectious triggers for conditions such as Alzheimer's and depression. Similarly, studies of the viral basis for multisystem disease in Covid long haulers might color how we research or think about lupus and connective tissue disorders, or multiple sclerosis and neurodegenerative disease.

"If we can help inform treatment of ME/CFS or autoimmunity, or any other diseases that are related, that would be my dream come true," Iwasaki said.

Chapter 9

THE NIH GOES BIG

In the first weeks of 2020, while patient advocate Alison Sbrana was running the two-week gamut of ME/CFS testing at the NIH, the scientists leading that study were preparing for the onslaught of neurological complications that would stem from the coronavirus.

Dr. Avindra Nath, the clinical director at the National Institute of Neurological Disorders and Stroke, has spent the majority of his career studying the intersection of infection and the brain, beginning with HIV in the 1980s. A professor at the University of Kentucky, and then at Johns Hopkins University, he joined the NIH in 2011. During the Ebola outbreaks in West Africa starting in 2014, he worked in Liberia, developing a patient cohort to look at Ebola's long-term neurological effects. He and his team had also been involved with researching the Zika virus, which spread from Brazil in 2015, as well as the tropical mosquito-borne Dengue fever. As the NIH upped its investment in ME/CFS, it tapped Nath to lead the study.

"We got involved with ME/CFS because a lot of these patients do complain of an infectious trigger," Nath said. "And the question really was, is it possible that there may be a persistent virus in the individuals and that may not disappear completely, or is it possible that it may just be an immune dysregulation?"

In 2016, he began building what was touted as perhaps the most detailed study ever of ME/CFS, performing extensive testing on a cohort of ME/CFS patients in an effort to isolate a common biomarker explaining the widespread types of suffering and unusual symptom patterns across the disease. Studies at the world's largest research hospital carried benefits, such as freedom from the constraints of private insurance companies regarding which tests could be done in a private hospital, as well as providing the funding to keep patients to study for weeks at a time. That type of robust approach to basic science carried the promise of finally cracking the medical enigma. After the last few years of poring over the sea of data from patients in the ME/CFS study, when Covid came along, Nath had a palpable sense of the overlap between the neurological conditions.

"We expected to see ME/CFS-like manifestations with these patients because we've seen it with all other infections," Nath said. "So we weren't that surprised, although I think we were surprised by the extent of involvement because it seems pretty severe." Persistent symptoms occurred at a much higher rate in Covid compared with Epstein-Barr virus, to which more than 90 percent of the population has been exposed. Thirty percent of the total population didn't report chronic Epstein-Barr complications. But as SARS-CoV-2 seemed poised to inexorably sweep through the majority of the human race, those significant rates of ongoing illness were showing up in some cohorts of Covid survivors.

Early in the pandemic, hospitals had set up post-Covid clinics to support patients recovering from acute respiratory distress syndrome, or ARDS, a form of lung failure that occurs when air sacs in the lungs fill with fluid. Severe Covid patients with ARDS couldn't breathe on their own and needed ventilators. After hospitalization, they had a lengthy road to recovery to heal their lung scarring and regain normal function. Instead, those clinics started filling up with patients who had never been admitted to intensive care and did not have the lung scarring.

The NIH, which commanded a nearly $43 billion budget in 2021, is largely known for doling out research funds to outside researchers. About 10 percent of its funding stays in-house, dedicated to nearly 6,000 scientists across its 27 distinct institutes and centers primarily located at its campus in Bethesda, Maryland.

One of the agency's most important functions—which occupies a little over half of its resources—is supporting *basic* research, delving into how organisms fundamentally function. Those kinds of studies look at how cells talk to each other or how genes are linked to specific traits. They may not appear to have any direct or immediate clinical human benefit, but they provide a vital scientific foundation for biomedical advances. Most major breakthroughs can be traced in some way to science done purely for science's sake. For instance, decades of molecular research into the immune system seeded immunotherapy in cancer. A study of how bacteria protect themselves from viruses ultimately led to the gene editing tool CRISPR, and its inventors, Jennifer Doudna and Emmanuelle Charpentier, won the Nobel Prize in Chemistry in 2020. And simple curiosity about mRNA, with little thought to future applications, eventually created the knowledge base that made it possible to build a Covid vaccine as soon as the virus genome was sequenced.

Basic science is invaluable to what experts call *applied* science, which is where the other half or so of the NIH's budget goes. Applied science focuses on practical solutions to real problems, looking directly at a disease itself. It is critical for *translational* science, where not only is the benefit to humans more obvious, but there are actionable ideas or interventions going from research lab bench to patient beside.

By October of 2020, the NIH had structured its Covid-19 research priorities into four distinct areas. First was developing a more robust understanding of the coronavirus. Second was studying therapeutics that could save the lives of those in the acute stages of Covid-19. Next was the all-important race to develop and distribute a vaccine that might end the pandemic. And the final major pillar of the nation's leading medical research agency was long haulers: how many were there, what subsets might they fall into, why were they sick, and what could be done to get them better? Scientists recognized that Long Covid was a crisis with devastating long-term ramifications.

Nath began giving presentations to colleagues at the NIH in which he explained the neurological complications and post-viral syndromes Covid-19 long haulers were developing. There was acute disseminated encephalomyelitis, acute necrotizing hemorrhagic encephalopathy, transverse myelitis, Guillain-Barré Syndrome, and dysautonomia. Finally, Nath's list included myalgic encephalomyelitis/chronic fatigue syndrome and dysautonomia.

SOLVING THE BILLION-DOLLAR QUESTION

Throughout the summer of 2021, the NIH laid the groundwork for its signature study for Researching Covid to Enhance Recovery, or RECOVER Initiative. The program embodied how it would address its pillar of focus around the long-term effects of SARS-CoV-2. While Congress had allocated nearly $1.2 billion for what it called the post-acute sequelae of Covid-19, or PASC, the bulk of the funding flowed through a massive "parent" award of nearly $470 million to New York University Langone Health, which would then delegate dozens of sub awards to about 100 researchers across more than 200 sites. The initiative was the largest systematic effort in the world to tackle Long Covid.

For those who had disabling symptoms a year and a half into the pandemic, the huge study was welcome, although it moved too slowly for people whose livelihoods were being destroyed by the long-term illness. Big announcements can generate positive headlines. But they're still a long way from final data or actionable results that can make a difference in daily experience, stemming the tide of a migraine or enabling a long hauler, in some cases, to just take a shower. Still, though, the NIH had managed to accomplish in a matter of six months what could usually be a two-to-four-year process for rolling out a study of such a scope, NIH director Francis Collins told press at the time.

During that development time, researchers had raced to create master clinical protocols so that all the institutions were following the same procedures, harmonizing data across all the sites so as to enable apples-to-apples comparisons among as many as 40,000 participants, with all researchers speaking the same language. A common scientific vernacular could avoid the pitfalls of small independently designed studies not fitting together into a comprehensive picture. Participants would need to represent every area of American life—including children, pregnant women, newborn babies, and the elderly—as part of a "meta cohort" pooling multiple groups of patients and controls together. They dedicated time to listening to patients, caregivers, and advocacy groups such as the Long Covid Alliance in an effort to create studies that met real human needs.

New York University Langone would handle the clinical science core, Massachusetts General Hospital would lead on tracking data resources, and the Mayo Clinic would host the biorepository managing specimens, making them available to researchers to study.

One of the problems that had plagued early research into Covid therapeutics was the proliferation of hundreds of small studies in which scientists chose their own pet drugs to test on their patients, each lab or institution acting independently, with no real battlefield general directing a coordinated attack on the disease. Some 92 percent of the trials attempted in the first year of the pandemic for acute Covid didn't reach completion or didn't report their results on ClinicalTrials.gov. Of the trials that were published, many were underpowered, without enough participants to achieve statistical significance. Many trials didn't include a randomized control group, so there was no way to determine if they outperformed a placebo. Depending on which end point a study measured—such as clearing the virus, discharge from hospital, or resolution of symptoms—studies could produce widely varying perspectives on whether interventions were effective or not. Moreover, because many hospitalized Covid patients eventually "recovered" anyway, it was hard to discern if a drug had actually saved a life or if the person's own immune system finally kicked in to clear out the raging virus. There had been breakthroughs, including monoclonal antibodies and results from a large UK trial showing that repurposing the corticosteroid drug dexamethasone could reduce risk of death. But in the first year and a half, those discoveries had been few and far between.

The world had bet big on the race to a vaccine, and as cases dwindled in the summer of 2021, the bet appeared to be paying off. There just hadn't yet been a similar emphasis on therapeutics for acute Covid, let alone Long Covid. The long haul took a back seat to the emergency.

"One critical way to prevent Long Covid is to prevent Covid itself," NIH director Francis Collins said during the House Energy and Commerce Committee hearing in April 2021. Preventing Covid meant getting vaccinated, wearing a mask, social distancing, and the whole litany of public health precautions that had become routine for most people during the pandemic. But, Collins noted, the agency was moving with "unprecedented" speed to fast-track treatments. That could mean anticoagulants for those with symptoms likely driven by blood clots, and steroid or immunosuppressants to drive down autoimmune reactions.

The command-and-control organization with which the RECOVER Initiative was designed could bring real systematic scientific rigor.

"People suffering now are a year out, going on two years out, and not getting better. So the time demand, the time urgency, is really turned up for this one. It begged for a more engineered approach," said Dr. Walter Koroshetz, the Director of the National Institute of Neurological Disorders and Stroke, and a co-chair of the RECOVER Initiative. "At the same time, we can't overengineer, so we have to be flexible. It may be a big surprise what's driving persistence."

In his role overseeing the NIH's neurological institute, Koroshetz had been involved in several recent multi-billion-dollar initiatives, including the Brain Research Through Advancing Innovative Neurotechnologies (BRAIN) Initiative, begun in 2013, which had plotted a twelve-year strategy to understand the human brain, transforming neuroscience in the way the Human Genome Project did for genetics. And he had co-chaired the Helping to End Addiction Long-term (HEAL) Initiative, which funded hundreds of research projects nationwide designed to end the opioid crisis by seeking new ways to treat pain and counter addiction.

"This one is much more focused," he said. "This one has one big trunk right now, then we're going to put the branches on, and have the trunk turn depending on where the science goes."

One key aspect of the RECOVER Initiative was the autopsy component, which would examine tissues under the microscope to find out where the virus could be hiding in ways that couldn't be done via a blood test or an imaging study. Autopsy studies open up incredible opportunities to learn about viral persistence in ways that can't be done in a living organism, particularly in whether or not the SARS-CoV-2, or its fragments, may have infiltrated parts of the brain.

The tens of thousands of people in the study would be grouped to compare those who recovered from acute infection with those experiencing persistent symptoms, along with a control group of participants who didn't get Covid. The effort also contained a major electronic medical records component to observe the health outcomes of millions of people over five or ten years following a Covid infection. It could look into whether the virus and their body's reaction to it would be linked to increased rates of diabetes, cardiovascular disease, or dementia. Collecting these massive amounts of data could bolster the case for how to pick the best drugs for clinical trials, and there was already a strong rationale to begin investigations into some therapies. But the process would take time, with the launch of new clinical trials estimated twelve to eighteen months away.

Nobody wanted this level of abject human misery, but if it had to occur, then systematically studying it was a massive opportunity to recast how we understand human immunology and what viruses can do to us. You didn't want the crisis to go to waste.

"This is a large natural experiment that offers the best chance to understand what happens to people with ME/CFS," Koroshetz said. "Here you know exactly when everybody got infected. You know exactly what the virus was. And you can actually study the recovery period. If you were going to put together an experiment to understand ME/CFS, this is exactly what you would design."

THE PATIENTS' VOICE IN STUDY DESIGN

Meanwhile, Karyn Bishof, the founder of the Covid-19 Longhaulers Advocacy Project and the co-founder of the Long Covid Alliance, was less sanguine about the likelihood of the massive initiative yielding important insights into the underlying causes of Long Covid or the soup of post-viral syndromes it caused. She was disabled by the dozens of Long Covid symptoms she felt every day, and she feared for her and her son's futures.

"It's ironic that for the whole pandemic it's been the patients educating the doctors and the research world, but for the development of this study, it felt as if nothing we said mattered," she said. "In my opinion, it is a waste of half a billion dollars that they are spending on this because the data that we've collected as patients tells us fifty times more than what they're gonna find through this. It's just really frustrating because I know that there is no help coming from this study."

She emphasized that no experts in ME/CFS or POTS, her most disabling diagnosis, participated in designing the study, a fact that other patients involved in the planning highlighted to me as well. She and other long hauler patient advocates felt like afterthoughts in the planning process. In the late summer of 2021, during the later stages of the RECOVER planning process, they'd received an email from the initiative's leadership team on a Friday night asking for six patients to appear in a weekend meeting.

"We had no idea what the meeting was for at all. We just clicked on the link to join the meeting when it started, and they just immediately jumped into talking about the study that they were designing," she said. "We were all like, 'What wait, like, what is happening? What are we doing?'"

The patient representatives had little time to coordinate among themselves, determine who felt strong enough to attend, or to plan which of them had the most useful expertise to share in any particular specialization of the research. They were unceremoniously split up into meetings with investigators across clinical specialties for various organ systems—problematic when nearly everyone experienced multisystem illness. As patient enrollment began across the nation, Bishof and other advocates weighed whether they ought to publicly lambast the plan, or to quietly acquiesce, so as to preserve slots on the patient advisory committees to try to influence the study as it progressed.

The Long Covid Alliance could boast a lofty-sounding name, an impressive list of hundreds of partners, and a status acting as a liaison for patients with Congress and federal agencies. But it didn't have paid staff members, or a traditional formal structure. With primarily sick volunteers, Long Covid advocacy groups didn't have the bandwidth for the tedious behind-the-scenes work of standing up a 501(c)3 non-profit organization. It takes years to build an effective fundraising apparatus and transition all of the grassroots advocacy into a formal office capable of building strong partnerships with huge institutions. And they were attempting this massive undertaking on the fly during a pandemic. That lack of resources or capacity meant triaging the most important tasks. Advocacy for the larger collective of long haulers necessarily took a backseat to one's basic day-to-day survival. But for many patients, particularly those like Bishof, calling for policy changes and simple self-preservation were inextricably bound together.

Harvard's Michael VanElzakker, long known within the ME/CFS researcher community as one of its most innovative thinkers, had submitted a research proposal for RECOVER but didn't receive funding. He expressed similar pessimism that the Long Covid crisis might go to waste.

"It *was* a once-in-a-generation opportunity," he told me. "I hope it isn't squandered. I hope we do make progress, but it's a little bit like saying 9/11 was a once-in-a-lifetime opportunity to have a new diplomatic regime. We had the sympathy of the world behind us. We could have said, 'Hey, let's right now become a humanitarian superpower.' It was a moment where a big shift could have happened but existing institutions tend to take advantage of opportunities like that, and promote their own sort of vision for things."

Instead, of course, the U.S. had doubled down with an aggressive foreign policy and wars in Afghanistan and Iraq. A medical equivalent might mean continued gaslighting and lack of treatment for those with complex chronic illness.

Comments such as VanElzakker's and Bishof's tore at me. They undermined my own premise as a patient, advocate, and journalist biased toward idealism and hope. I worried that just as the pandemic had exposed a myriad of inequities across society and nations, it had revealed massive unalterable weaknesses in how the healthcare system treats post-viral syndromes as well. And the question remains: will the agenda of big institutions drown out the most valuable stakeholders' contributions and squander our chances at substantial progress in the field of post viral illness? Or will determined and organized patients elbow their way to a seat at the table?

Mt. Sinai's David Putrino had worked hand-in-hand with patient communities to translate their experiences, broadcast treatment guidelines to thousands of clinicians through the American Academy of Physical Medicine and Rehabilitation and then made aggressive strides with a network of researchers to investigate the underlying physiology of the illness. His grant was denied. After he and his international colleagues had made some important findings about blood and inflammatory abnormalities in Long Covid, they chuckled to themselves: "Wouldn't it be great if we solved this without a cent of NIH funding?"

To him, it felt like the NIH was just an insular club, awarding grants to the same core group of researchers who had received them before in their respective fields. Putrino didn't feel they were asking the right questions because they weren't talking with the patient community or working with the community clinically. One grant that got the greenlight was $4 million for a study on high-intensity interval training.

If you consulted a Long Covid patient about the likelihood of that helping them, they would have said "Hell, no."

"Personally, I wish we had patient-led community members on the study sections evaluating the science," Putrino said. "I can't for the life of me understand why that is not happening. It should be happening. I think that in Long Covid it would be a very productive step and a very progressive step to take to include people like Body Politic to have a voice in who gets funded and doesn't get funded."

The NIH values incremental science, which can be very important in most areas. Scientists attending grant-seeking workshops are advised to explain how their new idea is an incremental step forward from the foundation of what's already known. In doling out taxpayer dollars, that type of conservative approach is necessary. They can't walk out like Oprah, saying, "You get a grant, and you get a grant!" But in the case of a novel illness, it doesn't work, and it's anathema to disruptive innovation that can deliver results that patients can use.

To Putrino, it seemed as though the people sitting on committees reviewing grants were just pushing their own line of research, campaigning to fit Long Covid into the box of what they had been studying prior to the pandemic, whether it was relevant to long haulers or not. Putrino lamented that the NIH system has not been patient-centered, patient-led, or even patient-involved.

"Why are you spending billions of dollars of taxpayer money and not asking us what we think as the people living with the condition? And that is a very reasonable question," he said. "It's condescending to assume that patients can't understand the science. No. Write it in a way that they can understand and you'll be a better scientist for it."

In November 2021, the Harvard T.H. Chan School of Public Health held a panel discussion on Long Covid moderated by Body Politic's Fiona Lowenstein and featured the Patient-Led Research Collaborative's Hannah Davis. The panel included Dr. Gary Gibbons, the director of the National Heart, Lung, and Blood Institute, and a co-chair of the RECOVER Initiative. Davis had pointed words for Gibbons, telling him that the NIH was "failing" in its patient engagement efforts, and long haulers' hopes for science to deliver them back to health were breaking. Gibbons asked for a follow-up meeting to hear their concerns and hash out how to address them.

Later that month, the PLRC published an open letter, co-signed by international patient groups for Long Covid, post-viral conditions, and dysautonomia. The letter issued a stark warning that "this initiative—which has raised the hopes of millions who are struggling with the myriad challenges of Long COVID even as the COVID-19 pandemic persists—is in grave danger of failing at its goals." At the top of the list were two fundamental concerns requiring structural adjustments to "safeguard the integrity and success of the initiative itself."

First, the patient representatives called for a "comprehensive and adequately resourced patient engagement structure." The PLRC gave a draft proposal for a rigorous plan based on best practices for how the NIH had partnered with HIV patients. For HIV, that partnership of patients, researchers, and government had only come about after activists had forced their way to the table. The same would likely be true for Long Covid as well. Though government agencies had lauded patient researchers' profound early contributions to researching and characterizing the condition, it now seemed to them as though the NIH was just paying lip service to the idea of patient engagement, treating them like tokens rather than collaborators.

Second, the PLRC called for post-viral illness experts to be "integrated into the Initiative, as well as supported as a collective advisory panel in the RECOVER structure." Seven months earlier, the Body Politic had urged the NIH to build its Long Covid study on the foundation already established by longtime researchers in post-viral illnesses such as ME/CFS, for which more than half of long haulers met the diagnostic criteria. However, patient representatives felt that the initiative's leadership only had a shallow understanding in the field of post-viral research, and the study would amount to just reinventing the wheel, ignoring the sprawling literature already available for ME/CFS, POTS, and mast cell activation syndrome.

Ensuring their voices were fully heard wasn't going to be a matter of any single meeting with any one official. It would inevitably be a project of many months, if not years, of entrenched, strident, and sophisticated advocacy. The pandemic survivors' quest to reclaim wholeness was informed by the history of social justice movements for women's rights, civil rights, and gay rights. They were propelled by knowledge from similar fights in the history of other diseases, the newest embodiment of abolitionist Frederick Douglass' statement that "power concedes nothing without a demand."

Chapter 10

GASLIGHTING, DISBELIEF, AND THE SEARCH FOR ANSWERS

WHEN SOMEONE IS *GASLIT* IT means that another person is trying to cause them to question the lived reality of their experience. The term has its roots in the 1944 film *Gaslight* starring Charles Boyer and Ingrid Bergman. The character Gregory, played by Boyer, spends the narrative attempting to manipulate his wife Paula, played by Bergman, into believing she is insane so that he can distract her from his crimes. One of his tactics is to cause the lights in the house to dim down and then to brighten again, which he does by turning on lights in their house's attic, diverting gas from the downstairs lights. He then tells her that the lights weren't flickering at all, but rather that it's just a figment of her imagination.

The concept of "gaslighting" as manipulation remained relatively obscure, mostly only to be talked about within the boundaries of psychology, until it experienced a renaissance as Donald

Trump ran for president and held office. Journalists began to widely use it to describe the ways in which the president's words and rhetoric departed from reality, often lying about basic facts. The term had become so prevalent that the Oxford University Press named it as a runner-up for the most popular new word in 2018. So, it was at the tip of the collective tongue in 2020 as long haulers reported lingering illness and doctors told their patients—predominantly women—that the symptoms were all in their head.

While the term is just gaining wide usage, the concept is not new to the medical community. A specific type of gaslighting, known as medical gaslighting, occurs when a medical professional dismisses a patient's complaints and insists their physical symptoms are imaginary. Discouraging at best, and life-threatening at worst, medical gaslighting happens disproportionately within disease clusters where diagnosis is challenging or complex. Furthermore, the propensity to minimize patient voices is exacerbated by medical racism and sexism. The effects of medical gaslighting can be devastating, resulting in post-traumatic stress disorder as one begins to question their own reality, and even death due to missed diagnoses. In fact, experts often refer to the recipients of gaslighting as victims of emotional abuse and see that they have the scars to prove it.

Women have been victims of this kind of malpractice for centuries. Ancient Greek medical texts dating to the fifth century BC attributed many of women's health complaints to a "wandering uterus" that needed to be controlled. By the seventeenth century, hysteria, derived from the Greek word for uterus, *hystera*, was considered a distinct physical disease common among women and tied to either their reproductive organs or their delicate nerves. In the late 1800s, after Sigmund Freud and the rise of psychoanalysis, a new prejudice was brewing as the cause of hysteria changed from the physical into the mental: hysterical symptoms began to be blamed on the patients' "unconscious mind." Make no mistake, the condition was still squarely seen as a women's ailment, but its roots were now thought to be in women's disordered psychology. It wasn't until 1980 that the diagnosis of hysteria was removed from the American Psychiatric Association's Diagnostic and Statistical Manual of Mental Disorders.

Despite the removal, the idea that women's unexplained physical symptoms are often "all in their heads" has persisted like a stain that resists cleansing. For millennia, hysteria was the metaphorical junk drawer where everything unorganized and unexplained was neatly kept without question or consequence. And, as journalist Maya Dusenbery argues in *Doing Harm: The Truth About How Bad Medicine and Lazy Science Leave Women Dismissed, Misdiagnosed, and Sick*, the concept continues to lead "to the persistent distrust of women's subjective reports of their own bodies—until those reports are backed up by objective evidence."

Fast forward to today, there is little intervention both in practice or medical training to combat systemic medical sexism, gender bias, and gaslighting. This reality has led to a system full of medical providers who undoubtedly hold implicit bias passed down through generations of oppressing women. This bias has found its way into the exam room, to the hospital bedside, and today leads to the dismissal of women's physical ailments. In one survey, 83 percent of women with chronic pain reported they felt they were discriminated against by their health care providers because of their gender. Research backs up these experiences, showing that women tend to experience longer diagnostic delays, wait longer for pain treatment, and often receive less treatment for the same maladies compared to their male counterparts.

Furthermore, women have historically been underrepresented in clinical research and many common conditions, such as heart disease, have historically been studied in cisgender male patients, under the assumption that the same conditions will present the same way in women. They often don't.

Women with a range of conditions often find that their symptoms are dismissed as depression, anxiety, or stress, before finally getting an accurate diagnosis after receiving proper testing. But for those with poorly understood conditions that don't yet have clear objective biomarkers, including post-infectious syndromes, this kind of medical gaslighting is often an ongoing part of the patient experience. While anxiety and depression often accompany the loss of control and suffering people encounter with physical disease, their reasonable and expected existence in the face of illness has confounded the casual relationship between the brain and the body. Through the lens of gender bias and long-held collective beliefs surrounding hysteria, when anxiety or depression are present, many doctors incorrectly assume they are causing physical symptoms.

In reality, the directional relationship between emotional symptoms and physical changes is often reversed. Emotional changes are frequently responses to factors such as physical changes in the brain due to the illness itself, the psychological toll that physical illness takes on a person, and loss of one's autonomy due to the disease. Emotional changes can also stem from provider gaslighting, a lack of a support system, and isolation due to physical constraints. All of these issues call on science and the medical community to persist in searching for the actual physical cause. For instance, while it's known that stress and emotions can influence physical health, in the case of heart disease, one would not reasonably suggest that heart disease is psychosomatic because of this relationship. The emotional toll of medical gaslighting is equally damaging as women question their own instincts and sanity in the face of authority while simultaneously battling painful physical symptoms and isolation.

Racial minorities are also at an increased risk of medical gaslighting. Researchers from the University of Virginia showed that Black Americans are undertreated for pain when compared to their white counterparts. In addition, the research showed that bias, whether implicit or explicit, was to blame and contributed to this unequal care. The study found that about half of the white medical students and residents held unfounded medical beliefs surrounding the biological differences between white and Black people (e.g., Black people's skin is thicker; Black people's blood coagulates more quickly, Black people age more slowly than whites, Black people's nerve endings are less sensitive than whites). A 2013 review published in the American Medical Association's Journal of Ethics suggested that the inequity in pain treatment across race was in part due to false held beliefs involving the motivations for pain medication, providers wrongly assuming Black and Hispanic people were more likely to abuse drugs. The racism found within the medical system presents a long, complicated, and stubborn problem. Some researchers now use the term "structural racism" to describe the multilayer issue at the core of health inequity among racial groups. This inequity, steeped in the historical oppression and exploitation of people of color, has understandably resulted in a mistrust in science and medicine in many communities of color. That mistrust has been exposed during the Covid-19 pandemic.

In her paper "The Sociology of Gaslighting," Harvard postdoctoral fellow Paige Sweet suggests that gaslighting "should be understood as rooted in social inequalities, including gender, and [is] executed in power-laden intimate relationships." In addition, she argues that "abstract social inequalities can be transformed into interpersonal weapons…when perpetrators mobilize gender-based stereotypes and structural and institutional inequalities against victims to manipulate their realities." And while there are many reasons and theories as to why it happens, we know the minimization of people's pain is a trend found within the entire American medical structure, but disproportionately so for minorities and women.

It was no surprise, then, that people well-versed in chronic illness worried that Long Covid might be dismissed by the medical community like the many complex ailments that came before it. They had seen this play before, and it frequently ended as a tragedy. In late 2020, however, even with the RECOVER initiative not yet in public sight, there were initial glimmers that this play might have a different ending. That hope rested in the development of a new type of Covid clinic, dedicated specifically to those with Long Covid. But not all that glitters is gold.

CASTING DOUBT ON GRADED EXERCISE THERAPY

The Long Covid clinics popping up across the world, and organized in the UK by the country's National Health Service, were by no means a quick fix for the illness.

The UK-based Long Covid Support organization ran a survey of 846 patients, which painted a portrait of a health system struggling to grapple with the longer-term health crisis it had now inherited. Claire Hastie, the group's founder, presented it to the UK government's Long Covid Roundtable in June 2021.

The patient group's survey showed that only a quarter of patients were satisfied with their experiences, and 58 percent felt dissatisfied. On the positive side, some people reported receiving thorough workups with doctors who listened carefully and empathized with their condition. For instance, one respondent reported coming away very impressed with their hourlong appointment, noting that "it felt like a collaboration," and received referrals to a cardiologist, respiratory therapist, and pain specialist.

However, a majority didn't feel they were receiving quality care. The survey revealed a range of complaints, the first of which was that it was hard to obtain a referral to access the clinic in the first place. Upon winning the referral to the clinic, wait times between seeing a general practitioner and the specialist were usually five to six months. Throughout the summer of 2021, as many clinics were still being set up, Hastie told me the wait times weren't improving, with some who'd first fallen ill in March 2020 still waiting for even a phone call from a Long Covid clinic. One sufferer in London complained of waiting "three months to get an appointment, then another two months to discuss my initial test results, then I was discharged so am now back in the exact same situation as I was prior to the first appointment."

In addition, the patients complained that many clinicians did not spend enough time with patients to get a grip on the full range of their complex symptoms. And some clinics appeared as though they'd been set up more as vehicles for research than as centers dedicated to quality care, collecting information about Long Covid symptoms but not providing those who were ill any guidance on how one might get their normal life back following months of illness.

"This is a sham service," one patient wrote after an appointment at a clinic in Bristol. "There is only a pretense at assessment before being shunted onto a rehab program that is designed for recovered Covid patients, not Long Covid. It is graded exercise, which they denied and offered in the full knowledge that I suffer [post-exertional malaise] and cannot exercise. Much as I respect physiotherapists, they should not be running a Long Covid service, as they are here."

The debate about whether graded exercise therapy helps in post-infectious syndromes is long and tangled. *Guardian* columnist George Monbiot found that out when he wrote a piece in January 2021 calling for massive research programs into Long Covid and similar illnesses. He argued that the population of the UK was on the precipice of a wave of long-lasting consequences from the pandemic, and letting the virus spread freely would exacerbate the effect, especially in the previously young and healthy.

Monbiot's column showed up the next month in a presentation that an Oxford psychiatrist gave to a large Swiss reinsurance company, a firm that provides insurance against major financial losses to other insurance companies. The psychiatrist specifically cited his article as an example of the "social factors" contributing to spreading the condition. According to the psychiatrist, news coverage of those with long-term symptoms served to hype up the illness, creating a hysteria that led many to become hypervigilant about their own signs and symptoms. Negative coping strategies along with too much focus on signs coming from their bodies became a vicious cycle that fed anxiety and depression. Online support groups, rather than serving as a validating lifeline in the midst of life-altering illness, were instead fertile soil for misinformation to grow.

Taken aback, Monbiot, a veteran investigative reporter, wrote a follow-up column headlined "Apparently just by talking about it, I'm super-spreading long Covid." It was like the proverbial question of the tree falling in the forest. Did Long Covid exist if there was no one there to write about it? "As I began to investi-

gate, I stumbled into one of the most astonishing scientific stories I've ever encountered," he wrote.

If Long Covid was psychogenic in nature, then it could be
meaningfully treated or cured by cognitive behavioral therapy
and graded exercise therapy. A mental health professional could
work with a client to treat an underlying depressive illness that
led to constant fatigue. At the same time, if fatigue and endurance problems were simply rooted in deconditioning, then grad-
ually building back one's exercise capacity would spark a return
to vitality. But many patients' everyday lived experiences, however, attested that this was false, as they would unavoidably crash
after minimal forms of exertion, such as walking up a flight of
stairs or cooking dinner. Years of research has shown post-exertional malaise as a cardinal feature of post-infectious diseases
such as ME/CFS. Why a post-exertional crash occurs in Long
Covid or ME/CFS is rooted in a relatively simple concept in exercise science. During a workout, a person's body burns oxygen to
convert it into glucose for energy. When she reaches her anaerobic threshold at a point of high intensity, her body switches to
a different process in which lactic acid is the byproduct—the
threshold is a point at which it becomes too strenuous to keep up
the pace and is tied to the level of muscle soreness the next day.
A strong athlete in a marathon might hit her anaerobic threshold
fourteen miles in. And while a healthy athlete may be sore after
a workout or even uncomfortable during it, hitting this threshold is a common process, and even a goal for some athletes in
order to increase stamina and build muscle. For someone with a
post-viral syndrome, it can take just a few minutes on an exercise
bike in a lab. And the more severely ill can hit the threshold just
after sitting on the bike seat before the test even starts. Once this
threshold is crossed for someone with exercise intolerance, the
person is now running on borrowed energy, and they will pay

for this with post-exertional malaise. Showing that this occurs is very doable. However, how and why it happens is a million-dollar question.

Rehab programs that push that type of patient to exercise beyond their anaerobic threshold are unsafe and can cause the disease to worsen, sometimes permanently, rather than improve.

Graded exercise therapy for ME/CFS had long been contentious, because it was based on the idea that the illness wasn't biological. Rather, the notion went, the symptoms were a result of patients forming false beliefs about their continued disability as their bodies became deconditioned, their minds mired in depression. Therefore, increasing exercise in successive increments every two weeks had appeared to be a logical way of affecting a full recovery, as pushed by the Oxford psychiatrists and similar proponents. And it could be combined with cognitive behavioral therapy that encouraged them to "challenge" a mindset grown accustomed to illness, with the patient's sickness supposedly motivated by a "secondary gain," which might include avoiding school or work, or obtaining drugs.

Such an approach can work well if the underlying notion of psychosomatic illness is correct, but it can be catastrophic if the illness is actually an organic and ongoing neuroimmune disease process, as it is in ME/CFS and Long Covid. The high-water mark for these treatment approaches had come in 2011 with the publication of the PACE Trial in *The Lancet*. At that point in time, the £5 million (about $8 million) study was the most expensive piece of ME/CFS research ever. Its findings have come to dominate clinical care for the disease in the UK and influence recommendations in the U.S. made by Mayo Clinic, Kaiser Permanente, and the CDC. The PACE Trial followed 641 patients in the UK and purported to show that graded exercise therapy could be recommended (the acronym refers to Pacing, graded Activity, and Cognitive behavior therapy: a randomized Evaluation). The study became mired in controversy, with surveys showing that patients felt graded exercise therapy harmed them, making their illness more severe in the long term. Patient organizations fought the recommendations. A report by the UK-based ME Association, published in 2015 and entitled "No decision about me without me," surveyed more than 1,400 patients and reached the conclusion that graded exercise therapy "should be withdrawn with immediate effect as a primary intervention for everyone with ME/CFS."

David Tuller, an investigative journalist and a public health academic at University of California at Berkeley who had reported on ME/CFS for years in publications including the *New York Times*, spent a year diving into the PACE trial. In 2015, he published a 15,000-word analysis disputing the study's methods on *Virology Blog*, a site run by a senior Columbia University microbiology professor. The piece helped galvanize a reappraisal of the exercise treatments, made all the more credible because Tuller holds a doctorate in public health.

But what was most remarkable was the way in which the whole story hinged on the abilities of patients to tell their own stories and assess data about their own disease themselves.

"When I wrote it, I made sure to say I was not some brilliant person," Tuller told me. "I got this from the patients."

Tuller leaned heavily on work by Tom Kindlon, a polite and mild-mannered Irishman who had been mostly homebound for two decades living with his parents, who were his caregivers, in the home in which he grew up. An avid athlete in his youth, Kindlon had played rugby, cricket, tennis, and soccer. But at age sixteen, Kindlon had caught some sort of bug during a hiking and sailing trip with friends in western Ireland. After recovering for a few days when he returned home, he found that after playing sports he totally crashed. By the end of his second year at Trinity College in Dublin, he could barely hold a pen in his hand. The disease forced him to permanently cut his math studies short in 1993.

Kindlon has a gift for statistical analysis. In his narrow bandwidth, studying scientific papers about the disease that had severely curtailed his life ambitions was the most obvious target of his passions. However, his abilities were very limited. In his forties, he could only stand for thirty seconds at a time before dizziness and balance problems forced him to lie back down.

Kindlon and other patients he met through online support networks "produced a sprawling online literature deconstructing the trial's methodology, submitted dozens of freedom-of-information requests for PACE-related documents and data, and published their criticisms on the websites and letters columns of leading medical journals," Tuller wrote.

Tuller argued that the trial was rife with flaws. For one, the researchers had used an overly broad definition of ME/CFS, such that a significant number of patients in the trial may not have had the actual disease. They also moved the goalposts after collecting data, lowering their definition of "recovery" to be far more inclusive. The study measured improvement based on subjective surveys. However, patient improvement in areas of objective measurements—such as whether they were able to return to work, get off disability, or if their fitness had improved—were so poor that they were ultimately dismissed as irrelevant or not objective after all. Tuller's investigation helped move forty-two scientists to sign an open letter to *The Lancet* calling for an investigation into the trial. Other scientists published their own independent critiques as well.

Meanwhile, in 2016, one patient won a court fight over his freedom of information request for PACE trial data that the investigators had not published. A three-judge panel ordered the sponsoring university to release the material. Patients and independent scientists who analyzed the data found that the likelihood that graded exercise therapy could help someone with ME/CFS was just 10 percent. And the likelihood it could lead to recovery was nil.

As biomedical research into the disease continued to amass, the notion that exercise could be a primary treatment strategy was failing to hold up. A 2015 report by the U.S. Institute of Medicine (now called the National Academy of Medicine) went as far as proposing to change the name of ME/CFS to "systemic exertion intolerance disease." If exercise intolerance was the primary feature of the underlying physiological disease, then prescribing a program of increasing exercise was about as counterintuitive as prescribing milk to someone who was lactose intolerant.

By 2017, the CDC dropped its recommendation for graded exercise therapy, updated its treatment guidelines to show that the disease could be made worse by exercise, and the U.S. federal Agency for Healthcare Research and Quality said there was no sufficient data to recommend the exercise treatment.

A similar evidence review published in the UK in October 2021 also confirmed the scientific consensus in favor of scrapping graded exercise as a primary treatment for ME/CFS, a decision that likely had reverberations for Long Covid. Published by the UK's National Institute for Health and Care Excellence—which sets treatment guidelines for the NHS—the new guidelines acknowledged that treating ME/CFS patients with fixed increases in exercise could cause harm if not conducted carefully as part of an individualized treatment plan. Patient groups, who had campaigned against mandatory exercise programs in NHS clinics for years, hailed the shift as the dawn of a new era in which the severe physiological underpinnings of the disease would be finally taken at face value.

They hoped the guidance, in the country that had been the home turf for the PACE trial, might help shift the culture in the country's Long Covid care centers where the coronavirus was causing ME/CFS-like illness, and have reverberations well beyond the UK border.

MAKING ROOM FOR CURIOSITY

Dr. David Lee, a researcher and emergency medicine physician at New York University Langone Medical Center, enrolled patients in a trial designed to test whether autoantibodies were driving POTS symptoms in Long Covid.

"I don't know if I can concretely say what works. I think the patients are honestly better at telling us what works and what doesn't," he told me.

Take, for instance, a concept such as "buzzing in the chest." It's not a symptom Lee had heard about in medical school, or that anybody had told him about, but patients reported feeling after Covid-19.

"Nothing pops into my head. So then, the only way to resolve that cognitive dissonance is to either say the patient's making it up—and that keeps my 'clinical experience' intact—or to say I don't have the clinical expertise for whatever this patient is feeling."

Threatened by mystery, and with minimal time for curiosity, many doctors can seem to reject a patient's lived experience if it doesn't fit treatment guidelines or a pre-existing mental schema. Lee felt some of the roots of that mindset could be traced to a technique in medical education referred to as "pimping," a brutal hazing technique that perverts the Socratic method of using thoughtful questions to guide students toward truth. When an attending physician "pimps" a trainee doctor, he baits the junior colleague to guess what he's thinking on some question of medical obscurity. Drawing a blank, or having failed to memorize an esoteric detail, means one's fund of knowledge is deficient. The pressure for a right answer, or at least any answer that *isn't wrong*, instills a fear of making a mistake and discourages a mindset in which mistakes can be embraced as an opportunity to learn.

Pimping has an obvious derogatory connotation of sex trafficking or prostitution in wider society everywhere outside the medical profession. A 2019 article in the journal *BMC Medical Education* argued the practice was "a tradition of gendered disempowerment" and called for it to end.

INTERSECTIONS OF DISBELIEF

If having a debilitating condition that's poorly understood by medical science isn't already difficult enough, having Long Covid as a Black woman adds another layer of struggle, compounding what we know about the history of medical neglect and mistrust among communities of color.

Cynthia Adinig, a thirty-four-year-old graphic designer from Alexandria, Virginia, got sick on March 20, 2020. Not long after, she joined the Long Haul Covid Fighters group on Facebook. The members exchanged research papers characterizing past pandemics. They found recent studies of post-Ebola survivors, suggesting that most of them got better after six months, and at first hoped that would be their illness trajectory as well. But the idea of recovery after Covid was a mirage for many of them.

"You could see the panic, and the grieving." she said. "It became clear that long haul meant *long haul*. It was like whoa, whoa, whoa, whoa, are we all gonna die? And that's one of the things we talk about a lot in the group, like is this a ticking time bomb? Are we waiting to die? Is there going to be a mass die-off however many months down the road, because our body is so wrecked?"

Chronic illness, though, doesn't necessarily finish off its victims, prompting harder questions about enduring a future of pain and suffering.

"There is but one truly serious philosophical problem, and that is suicide," Albert Camus wrote in 1942. "Judging whether life is or is not worth living amounts to answering the fundamental question of philosophy."

The problem of suicide is also a daily question for many of those in Long Covid support groups.

"If I can't form sentences, I'd rather not live." Adinig told me.

Her sister had died prior to the pandemic, leaving her mother depressed for about a year and a half, at times becoming suicidal. Adinig wouldn't tell her mother how severely Covid was affecting her for fear of adding to her already sizable emotional burden.

"I didn't die because I know it would, like, *break* her, break her. I made sure to live to make sure that she lived."

While sitting, out of nowhere she could feel a sensation she referred to as "The Climb," her heart rate rising up from normal to the range of 150 beats per minute. It was as though she were in a brisk run rather than simply sitting still. She had to relearn how to walk twice and didn't know if she could live with the privilege of being able to predict what she could accomplish from one day to the next.

"I used to go to sleep every night for well over a year, without knowing I was going to wake up," she said.

She developed violent food allergies, which restricted her diet to only four main foods: eggs, black beans, corn, and chicken, all prepared plainly with no spices. Anything else triggered significant reactions. Covid's assault on her body damaged her esophagus, leading to an esophageal tear that made it painful every time she swallowed. That, as well as her mast cell activation problems, triggered starvation and dehydration. Then those conditions, in turn, could spike her heart rate, exacerbating her problems with POTS.

"Grieving that old life was really, really rough," she told me. "I may have had my last birthday with a birthday cake and ice cream. I may have had my last holiday of turkey and macaroni and cheese. And I didn't know that. I may have had my last New Year with eggnog, and I may have had the last meal that I'll make for my child. It's not just that I can't eat food, I can't be around cooking. So that means I may have had my last visit to a restaurant. I may have had my last visit to a family gathering. And Black and Brown families rely *heavily* on food for family gatherings. If I could turn back time, I would have way more banana bread."

Beyond just having a debilitating disease, Adinig described forms of medical racism. She felt disbelieved due to the color of her skin and was drug-tested at an emergency room more than once.

"When the medical system discards us like trash and abuses us, it feels like rape. And as a victim of rape, I know what that feels like. Honestly it feels like that. When you have someone of power steal your trust, and then you're powerless to do anything, that to me is rape. I don't say it lightly, but that's what it feels like. It's that traumatic to continue to know that you need help, that the system you rely on to do the right thing for your body...I have no choice but to trust that they will care for me. To constantly have to give trust to your abuser for the sake of your life, that's a traumatic experience."

As horrifying as it was, she understood her experiences weren't uncommon and were downstream effects in a larger scope of history in which previous generations of Black people had been treated even worse.

"Our ancestors want us to persevere," she said. "They did not get through slavery for us to be brought down by gaslighting. They did not pick all the cotton, they did not survive all those beatings, just for me to be so mentally destroyed by the medical system to just say that I give up. I will never. I will never."

She vowed to do as much as she could to drive change on a broader scale, while living with the fact that she didn't know how much time she had left.

Advocates connected her to her local congressman, Rep. Don Beyer. She helped advise his legislative team as they constructed the Long Haulers Act, a $93 million piece of legislation with appropriations across several federal health agencies. As a political nerd, she had a hobby of reading Supreme Court cases, and considered legislation her happy place.

"I gave it a nice Black set of eyes," she told me.

Chapter 11

CHRONICLES
OF UNCERTAIN
RECOVERIES

MANEESH JUNEJA IS A CONSULTANT and speaker from London. The self-described "Digital Health Futurist" and former data manager for drug maker GlaxoSmithKline had expected to spend 2020 as he usually did: crisscrossing continents and advising governments and companies on health innovation. But he caught the respiratory illness on April 10, and Long Covid left him mostly bedbound for more than a year.

The disease caused him extraordinary fatigue, post-exertional malaise, and brain fog, as it does in many. But for Juneja, it also came with a bizarre feature in which if he tried to squat down to pick something off the floor, he couldn't pick himself up again and would fall over backwards. And it presented with an intense all-consuming pressure in his head. "It literally would last the whole day and it wouldn't be resolved in any way, and I'd often spend the whole day just wanting to cut my head open with a knife to release the pressure," Juneja told me.

He tracked his vitals using his Apple watch. On his finger, he wore an Oura ring, a smart device that tracks indicators such as sleep and how many calories one is burning. And every day Juneja doggedly tweeted out an update about his symptoms.

"I felt like I was doing something, like I was contributing to society or being of service whilst being sick, in that my tweet helps someone take the virus seriously, like, 'Oh my God, I don't want to get the virus in case I get Long Covid, because I can see what Maneesh is going through,'" he said.

His meticulous real-time accounting amassed an impressive public record of living through the disease.

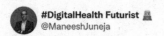

#DigitalHealth Futurist
@ManeeshJuneja

Day 105 of life with post #covid19 symptoms and I'm feeling **ok-ish** this morning. Here's a thread about yesterday's experience of getting 3 MRI scans done as part of my self funded investigation checking for damage to my body as a result of the virus #longcovid 1/n

11:37 PM · 7/21/20 · Twitter Web App

4 Retweets **23** Likes

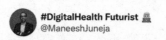

#DigitalHealth Futurist
@ManeeshJuneja

I'm literally **crying** tears of joy right now.

This is the first day in 197 days of #LongCovid that I have no symptoms at all, and feel completely normal in body and brain.

6:24 PM · 10/22/20 · Twitter for Android

4 Retweets **4** Quote Tweets **150** Likes

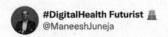

#DigitalHealth Futurist 🏛️
@ManeeshJuneja

Day **222** of #LongCovid - Whilst I seem to have emerged from my relapse, my health status is quite wobbly, so even more self compassion today.

1st time in 4 days I've had the mental & physical energy to take a shower!

It might sound trivial, but it brought me a lot of joy 🛁💦

1:50 PM · 11/16/20 · Twitter for Android

2 Retweets **93** Likes

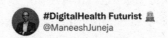

#DigitalHealth Futurist 🏛️
@ManeeshJuneja

Day **287** of living with #LongCovid & today's visit to a NHS Long Covid clinic was bizarre

The doctor was very dismissive of my symptoms, didn't believe I ever had covid (WTF!) and told me I was "very anxious"

Was then seen by a physio who "LISTENED" & didn't belittle me!

3:51 PM · 1/20/21 · Twitter Web App

47 Retweets **26** Quote Tweets **325** Likes

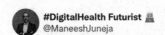

#DigitalHealth Futurist 🏛️
@ManeeshJuneja

It's now been 5 months since I had any kind of #LongCovid symptoms 😊

I still consider myself fully recovered

My brain and body continue to function normally without any **impairments**

A 🏛️ on my ongoing journey back to optimal health

1/n

8:04 AM · 9/20/21 · Twitter Web App

6 Retweets **5** Quote Tweets **121** Likes

Courtesy of Maneesh Juneja

One doctor wrote him, "As a GP, I've found your threads where you share the experiences you've had with your GP eye-opening and hugely helpful. It's changed the way I look at things and I hope it means I'm supporting patients better."

To paint a more vivid portrait of his experience, Juneja shared his tracking data from his smart devices with his general practitioner in the UK's National Health Service. He also conveyed the crowdsourced wisdom he'd received from others, so the doctor and patient could make informed decisions together as equals.

"Because of my activism and advocacy—because I've plugged in, because I'm literally looking at the data, the literature, the guidelines—I was able to guide her when many patients wouldn't have the resources or the literacy to guide their GP. And the GP can't say, 'Sorry, I don't know how to refer you to a clinic. Bye.'"

Juneja's doctor had no idea how to refer him to one of the NHS's brand new Long Covid clinics, which began coming online around six months into the pandemic. Having done all his research ahead of time, he coached her through the process, as she was overwhelmed by the demands of primary care and the onslaught of new research coming out.

"Here's the *patient* coming through steering for how to provide best care for the patient, and at times I felt like I was doing the doctor's job when the system wasn't giving her the resources to be able to do a proper doctoring job," he said.

Of course, patients shouldn't have to do professional-level research by diving into reams of peer-reviewed literature to replace a physician's role. But simply monitoring best practice collaboratives can raise one's level of awareness without needing to become a totally self-taught expert in one's own right.

For instance, when the CDC released their guidelines for post-Covid conditions in the U.S., they delivered patients a form of power they hadn't had before. Here was a document with the

CDC's logo on it that said that Long Covid was real. Patients didn't need a positive PCR test to be entitled to post-Covid care, and doctors should be able to make a Long Covid diagnosis based on one's symptoms and not rely solely on any single objective diagnostic test. In a situation where there's a shade of doubt about a patient's illness, guidelines such as those become crucial extra leverage for an informed patient to navigate effective care.

Juneja was educated on the NHS's policies, but getting into the clinic didn't help. The months of waiting for a so-called Long Covid "expert" proved to be false hope. The physician he was placed with, a respiratory specialist, dismissed his neurological complaints and the feeling of his head exploding with pressure as Juneja just being "hypervigilant." Juneja had gotten much more validation from the ME/CFS patients who'd commented on his tweets to tell him his pain was real, and the head pressure was a regular feature in their post-viral lives.

"I was so flabbergasted," he said. "I didn't even have the time to say 'WTF, I'm walking out of here.' That Long Covid clinic, if it was a private clinic, if I had paid to see the physician, I would have asked for my money back."

Still, Juneja eventually recovered, though he couldn't be sure if that could be attributed to two Pfizer jabs jumpstarting his immune system, the natural passage of time, adapting a lifestyle of intermittent fasting, or some other unknown reason.

What he does know is that becoming a patient shifted his perspective in how he works to design the future of digital health.

"What if you are diagnosed with an illness, and the healthcare system routinely signposts you to peer support groups, online and offline?" he suggested. "Not only that, but also signposts you to services where you can maybe have like a WhatsApp buddy who was also living with the illness, or a WhatsApp support group? Why can't the healthcare system of the future integrate with these groups?"

The process of elevating patient wisdom in a healthcare system could also naturally work as a release valve relieving pressure on doctors expected to be omniscient.

"Why can't we as patients be compassionate toward doctors?" he said.

Someone has to be the first to extend the olive branch across the patient-doctor aisle, and it may have to be the patients themselves.

RECLAIMING HER STORY

What are you, O great Mountain?

Those words from the fourth chapter of Zechariah fueled Mara Gay through the long and uncertain aftermath of Covid. In the verse, God speaks to the leader of Jerusalem with encouragement to rebuild the temple against great odds, offering to flatten mountains to aid the effort.

Gay's journey began in March 2020, when it felt as though she could hear her entire New York apartment block coughing. Alone and sick, she prayed for her neighbors. At age thirty-three, she was living her dream as a member of the *New York Times* editorial board and a political analyst for MSNBC. Her work abounded with purpose as she wrote editorials endorsing local candidates for office to lead her city. She hoped to get married, buy a house, raise children, and write a book.

The virus nearly killed her.

"You just take a deep breath and stop halfway," she said. "Then live that way for a year and a half."

After weeks of slow recovery, despite her shortness of breath, she had returned to running—not marathons, but a couple of miles at a time. Then, five months after the infection, out of nowhere, she had symptoms similar to those of a stroke and was admitted to the ER. She had what she would later learn were laryngeal spasms. The sensation—like a charley horse choking her on the inside of her throat—was diagnosed as what's called functional globus. It left her throat in such a state of inflammation that she couldn't talk for more than ten minutes at a time, or she would have to lie quietly on her stomach for an hour doing breathing exercises.

The virus had affected her nervous system.

"I don't want to say that I was suicidal because I didn't have any plans to kill myself or end my own life," she said. "But there were many moments where I thought if this is as good as it gets, I don't want to keep living in this body."

She credited her ongoing recovery to a combination of luck, genetics, physical therapy, time, prayer, health insurance, acupuncture, osteopathy, psychotherapy, friends, running, and her bosses allowing her to take three months off from work.

And "just sheer fucking determination."

"I don't blame doctors for this, but clinical medicine has done nothing for me," she said. She had seen three pulmonologists, two ENTs, two primary care doctors, four physical therapists, and a craniosacral therapist. When conventional doctors had nothing to offer, her skill as a reporter helped her navigate toward experts capable of treating her. While she appeared to be back to living a normal life, the reality was that she was still like a healthy person recovering from an injury. Every doctor who had examined her felt she would recover but it wasn't clear if that timeline might be two years, three years, or more. Gay leaned heavily on her Christian faith, which stemmed from her time organizing with the Black church while a student at the University of Michigan. The church's teaching, along with her humanism, fused together in her spirit. Listening to Martin Luther King, Jr.'s sermons built in her a justice-oriented spirituality. Faith was a practice for resisting real-world oppression. And that was made all the more relevant during the Trump administration, the pandemic, and her own illness.

"I believe that if I had known what Donald Trump knew about Covid when he knew it, I would not have ever gotten sick," she said. "We had a fascist president in the White House who was racist and didn't care about people who live in cities and who look like me."

Unable to draw a full breath for a year and a half, she came to see her life with Long Covid framed in the larger tide of history. Gay's grandfather was orphaned as a child when his father had died of treatable tuberculosis, unable to get care because he was Black. Similar dynamics abetted the virus and its complications in sweeping through communities of color.

The disease brought her closer to God.

"God, thank you that you've got this," she would pray. "I can't see a way, but I know you have a way. Thank you for going before me."

In her journey to reconcile her own healing with that of the nation, she found respite in Desmond Tutu's *The Book of Forgiving*. In it, the Nobel Laureate and architect of South Africa's post-apartheid healing process wrote that forgiveness isn't about forgoing justice. Rather, it's about reclaiming that which was stolen from you, removing yourself from being a victim, and rebecoming the author of your own life story.

"You can't be living in sickness in your head all the time," Gay said. "You're a survivor and you get to tell your story. Nobody gets to tell that story but you. Not the virus. Not other people. And not doctors."

Chapter 12

PRECURSORS: ME/CFS AND LYME

IN THE PRACTICAL REALITY OF running her clinic day to day, Dr. Nancy Klimas treated many Covid long haulers who presented just like the complex patients she was used to seeing for more than three decades. To be sure, there might have been some selection bias from long haulers who sought her out as an established ME/CFS expert, and then even more specifically as a physician who had a specialization in clinical immunology. But it was as though she was treating the same disease.

"In my practice, the immunology looks very similar: poor natural killer cell function, pro-inflammatory cytokine expression, immune activation, and immune exhaustion. Markers on flow cytometry are also very similar to what we'd see in ME/CFS," said Klimas, the director of the Institute for Neuro-Immune Medicine. "I think it's a reasonable hypothesis that we're going to see a lot of similarities between the two."

In short, the long haulers fit a description not unlike what Klimas had begun publishing about in the early 1990s, which was at the heart of her institute's focus on a variety of complex neuroimmune conditions, including fibromyalgia, Gulf War syndrome, Lyme, autism, and HIV/AIDS. The demographic profile also tended to be more female—likely, she believed, due to the fact that many inflammatory and autoimmune diseases tend to be more common in women. The biggest difference was that here there was an obvious viral culprit, and it might still be persistent in the body.

In the fall of 2020, the CDC tapped Klimas and her institute to be cartographers for this new post-Covid terrain, partnering with the clinician and her team in a $4 million study contract designed to understand the depth and breadth and severity of Long Covid. "I'm so excited with all these years of doing ME/CFS work and feeling like I've been dealing with a clinically biased population that I'm finally able to do this better design and really answer some important questions," she said.

But guiding that inquiry during a pandemic held its own challenges.

"We had a hard time getting this study off the ground because we had to build all these relationships with these healthcare systems, which turned out to be difficult," she told me. "Doable, but difficult." The process was a bit of a crash course in the overall fragmentation of the U.S. healthcare system, which makes it difficult to collect data efficiently. Countries with national health systems, such as the UK, have an advantage in producing better monthly statistics about Long Covid. Eventually the CDC study would reveal whether there are differences in the risk of long-term illness in those who were vaccinated versus those who weren't, and across the different variants of SARS-CoV-2.

They began by looking for people who experienced acute Covid-19 in the three to six months prior to enrollment. From there, the CDC and Klimas' team began longitudinally tracking 800 patients—200 who recovered, and 600 who remained ill. They are performing comprehensive testing looking at autonomic measures, biologic workups, and immune panels, comparing people who regained their health with those who remained ill, looking to determine the overall epidemiology of the disease and general profiles of who gets Long Covid. Their team, based in Fort Lauderdale, Florida, built a system to specifically recruit patients from the major healthcare systems in south Florida.

Deeper into the pandemic, in the winter of 2021, the mysteries were compounding. Were there any discernible differences in a person's Long Covid risk among the Delta, Omicron, and the original Alpha strain of the coronavirus? And while it was clear that vaccines and boosters were protective against severe illness and death, there weren't yet definitive answers on how well they could guard against Long Covid, given that most long haulers got sick following a mild infection.

One UK study showed that vaccinations could cut the risk of contracting Long Covid in half. That's good news. But when the virus is spreading in massive waves of up to a million cases per day in the U.S.—as it was in December 2021—there's little consolation in that data.

"Long Covid prior to Delta was not predicted by the severity of infection. We're seeing that over and over and over again," Klimas said. If the general rate of long-term symptoms is usually cited in a range between 10 percent to 30 percent in most studies, then halving the risk still means the rates of possible long-term illness might tally 5 percent to 15 percent. It's a mass disabling event, with a virus that can cause memory loss in young people wildly on the loose.

Breakthrough cases weren't uncommon during the Delta wave. And throughout the Omicron wave, vaccines largely prevented severe disease, but mild breakthrough cases were rampant. During the first wave, any Covid infection had some risk of triggering long-term symptoms. The same true is with Omicron, and subsequent waves of infection thereafter. Some of the most important—and most basic—questions about Long Covid proved unanswered even two years into the pandemic.

"It's going to be awful. There's going to be a lot of people sick for a long, long time because we already have a million people ill with ME/CFS, and we don't know what to do with post-infectious ailments," she said. "The potential that Long Covid is a likely second pandemic is extremely alarming when there is a political policy response right now that is arguing for herd immunity, letting everybody get infected. Certainly in my state that is widely said out loud."

BUILDING A FIRMER FOUNDATION

While Klimas was launching her epidemiology study with the CDC, the National Institutes of Health's RECOVER Initiative was starting to enroll thousands of patients around the country. Many Long Covid patient activists worried that that RECOVER Initiative might just rediscover the same types of post-viral abnormalities that Klimas and the coterie of neuroimmune experts had been finding for years, rather than launching off from the base they had so painstakingly assembled "on a whisper and a prayer." However, the base of knowledge—useful as it was for informed patients comparing notes in online communities—had never grown strong enough to truly fly the nest into the mainstream of medical practice.

"I have no problem with learning it all over again," Klimas said. "That's not a problem, particularly with this very well-funded group with a cohort of 15,000 people." As a leader in the post-viral field, she knew the prevailing themes in how patients could present with a range of immunological abnormalities, how persistent infections could often be at the root of the problem, and how imaging studies had shown neuroinflammation in the brains of those with ME/CFS. Despite the thousands of published research articles, though, most of the studies over the past thirty years were underpowered, conducted using small cohorts of a few dozen patients. A big study, by ME/CFS standards, might have 100 subjects in it. The studies were underpowered because they were underfunded, and it became impossible to repeat them at the larger scale needed to rewrite the medical textbooks. When researchers received funding, it was usually incumbent on them to show how their research might innovate in the field, to forge new ground, rather than to go back and validate an earlier finding.

So Klimas was elated to see how the NIH's call for research proposals had prompted hundreds of applicants from nearly every major university and health system. Teams were falling over themselves to submit grant applications to study Long Covid. It made her recall how when bank robber Willie Sutton was asked why he robbed banks, he replied, "That's where the money is." The same was now true for post-viral illness. The urgency to study the massive health crisis required narrow deadlines, with just twenty days between the application releasing until the day it was due, a process her team usually would have needed six months to accomplish. "When they put aside enough money to fund a small nation, then all of a sudden everybody went for it and had a deep burning interest in what was going on in these long-term ill Covid patients," she said.

And it wasn't just for the observational research delving into the underlying biology. Klimas was heartened that by late 2021 the NIH opened applications for researchers seeking funding for clinical trials to treat Long Covid. That stood in stark contrast to the titanic struggle to which she was accustomed with ME/CFS.

"Really? It's been thirty years and we've never had a program announcement that let us move to trial?" she said.

She had seen this sort of scientific sea change before. As a clinical immunologist, Klimas had worked early in her career treating HIV patients during the 1980s. That field of researchers started small with, at least at first, everybody knowing everybody else. One year there might be 500 attendees at the annual HIV research meeting at the Hilton in Washington, D.C. The next year, perhaps 800. But then the NIH invested massively in the research, and 10,000 people showed up at the conference.

You couldn't move your arm in the crowd without spilling someone else's drink. "Everybody in the room had coffee stains down their shirts," she laughed. "We were all standing with our elbows tight against our sides, moving through posters and exhibits with our coffees and our teas. Everyone looked like they had their coffee thrown at them." Of course, a little extra for a dry-cleaning bill was a tiny price to pay for catalyzing interest in solving the AIDS pandemic. But through the 1990s and 2000s, as Klimas focused her immunology career on a different set of acquired immune deficiency syndromes, there was less of a need to fight crowds. Her research team was among only a handful of teams in the country that routinely pulled down grants from the NIH to study ME/CFS and its cousin, Gulf War syndrome. Though they protested that the research field would grow directly if the funding levels grew, the message from federal agencies always seemed to be that funding levels should stay low because most scientists just weren't interested. It was a chicken or egg problem. But now the egg was finally cracking.

With Long Covid funding approaching major league levels, the interest from researchers at an annual meeting might again fill a large conference space, buzzing with new scientists spilling coffee on each other…assuming in-person meetings become advisable again. "It's an exciting and wonderful thing that this huge amount of money is going to be spent on this important study, I'm really behind it," Klimas said. "I'm just bemoaning the fact that it took a pandemic to get the interest in post-viral illness to the point where there's sufficient funding."

She had a wish list of drugs that she had been using with patients off-label for years and which could easily be slotted in for drug trials.

First, it was a chance to finally use antivirals in a definitive way. Some antivirals could work on both herpesviruses and coronaviruses, so even if the exact underlying mechanism wasn't clear, patients still might feel better and that was fine with her. "I'm sure it would be more mechanistically pure if you used a very, very specific coronavirus antiviral or very, very specific herpesvirus antiviral to try to discern these things," Klimas said. But overall, a drug might show efficacy even if it was closely, if not perfectly, targeted. From there, it would be important to try specific immune modulation drugs that could enhance cytotoxicity, the ability of immune cells to kill off invaders. Researchers ought to also try cytokine therapies that inhibit proinflammatory cytokines, such as Enbrel and Humira. Those three categories of therapies, she explained, had all shown some amount of success in ME/CFS in early phase clinical trials but hadn't received funding to move forward into the larger trials necessary to gain FDA approval.

Another broad area is drugs that repair patients' bioenergetic pathways. They would carry the virtue of being very safe and fast launching points following a "first, do no harm" philosophy. And those types of treatment studies could be launched inexpensively and remotely, without needing patients to come into the clinic, or live anywhere near the site.

Assuming sleep is distorted in Long Covid in the same way that it's disrupted in ME/CFS, then it follows suit that people have adrenaline surges at night that keep them up and have trouble balancing the sympathetic and parasympathetic nervous systems. "Restorative sleep is a very reasonable target and a very easy thing to survey to see if people are waking up feeling rested or not," Klimas said. "It's something that we routinely do in our clinic-based population and something we are doing in our CDC study. We should know a little bit more about the nature of sleep in this post-Covid illness and then interventions can be applied."

Ultimately, it would amount to a moonshot mission to cure the disease(s), and not just manage the symptoms.

CORONA WITH A TWIST OF LYME

Mark Twain reputedly said, "History doesn't repeat itself, but it often rhymes."

The notion is at once comforting and disturbing—that we're part of some unfolding song, that deeper patterns direct the uncertainty of our existence, that everything new in our collective experience resonates with something that's come before.

With each expert and patient I spoke to, I couldn't help thinking of how diagnosing and treating Long Covid felt so similar to controversies in the history of Lyme disease. It surfaced many of the same nagging questions. Were chronic cases driven by a persistent infection? Did symptoms emerge from a permanently altered immune system? How could people get so sick, and yet their underlying signs of disease be so difficult to detect? Could the infection reach into the brain? And why did this happen more commonly in women?

The fundamental questions pulled at me because in one version of events, my entire history of relapsing symptoms revolved around the tick-borne illness and the contested science around it. Growing up with one foot always in the woods, I'd constantly been exposed to ticks, regularly picking the little arachnids off the skin of my beloved black Labrador, Jenny. They showed up on my own skin as well.

But one bite haunted me. During a weeklong Boy Scout summer camp at age fifteen in Kentucky, I'd stopped by the little first aid hut with a tick stuck at the base of my left buttock. I couldn't twist far enough down to get a good look at it and remove it myself, so I asked the nurse to pry it off with tweezers.

"I got most of it," she told me. "But I couldn't remove the head."

I felt a little pang of panic in the pit of my stomach. Leaders constantly preached to Scouts the need to fully remove a tick—head and all. I knew those facts like a religious dogma, and violating them felt wrong. But the nurse was an authority figure and I just assumed it wouldn't matter.

For me, taking huge risks and testing rules was the point of camp in the first place. I instigated other boys in ramming sailboats until they submerged in the lake, and we occasionally sparked balls of fire in the air when cooking with propane stoves. So, taking a risk with a fragment of a bug—even one that caused a disease I was supposed to be afraid of—felt less ominous than a more obvious tragedy like a mishap on the shotgun range. Knowing little else I could do, I shrugged off the botched tick removal by the end of the week.

The bite site stayed red and inflamed for the next year. When all-consuming fatigue forced me to stop attending school, I showed the bite site to each doctor in the failed parade of diagnosis toward chronic fatigue syndrome. Each agreed it looked inflamed but my skin didn't match with the classic bullseye rash—a red splotch with a ring around it—characterizing most Lyme infections. And their blood panels showed I was negative for Lyme, according to the CDC's surveillance definition for the disease, which tests for specific antibodies to the infection.

Two years later, I found Dr. Bullington—my current doctor—and she ordered a more specific test offered through IGeneX, a California-based laboratory specializing in tick-borne diseases. Through its more expanded threshold for bands of detectable antibodies, I came up positive.

She explained to me that the mainstream methods for detecting Lyme may miss more than half of cases, according to one study.

From there, at least part of the strange years-long illness shifted into a clearer focus, potentially traceable to a discrete event in space and time.

Bullington added a course of long-term antibiotics to my already robust treatment plan. But because I was prescribed so many drugs and supplements at the same time, it's hard to know whether it was the antibiotics or prescriptions for other symptoms and abnormalities that had the greatest effect in my recovery. My health trended overall toward stability. Outside of torturous flare-ups here and there, the overall treatment plan built space for the pursuits that fulfilled me: I joined a college intramural soccer team, challenged myself academically with advanced astronomy and Mandarin Chinese, pursued love, and built a life.

After the antibiotic course, we drew blood for a Lyme culture test, which seeks to grow the bacteria in a lab over a period of weeks. Though it hasn't yet gained mainstream acceptance, the culture test, I was told, could definitively determine whether bacteria still existed in the blood, looking beyond whether the patient was capable of mounting an immune response.

At the time, I knew little about the decades of controversy around Lyme and tick-borne diseases, learning as much science as suited me through doctor's appointments, books, and Internet searches. But my own body was nothing if not a single data point in a vast scientific debate, one which lent yet another tantalizing lens through which to examine how we contend with the Covid and its long shadow.

Lyme disease is named for a cluster of cases in children and adults that appeared around the town of Lyme, Connecticut in 1975. Six years later, researchers linked the infections to the *Borrelia burgdorferi* spiral-shaped bacteria, or spirochete, which is carried by ticks. However, the disease has likely circulated for thousands of years. Researchers discovered parts of the *Borrelia* genome in the prehistoric mummy Ötzi, also called Ice Man, who was preserved in the Alps between Austria and Italy after likely being murdered some 5,300 years ago.

In the days or weeks after a tick bite, acute Lyme most often appears with the bullseye rash alongside fever, chills, fatigue, and muscle and joint aches, according to the CDC. It has reached epidemic levels, and today the agency estimates there are 300,000 new cases—or possibly even more—of Lyme each year in the U.S., with 10 to 20 percent of those infected remaining ill after treatment.

Lyme has been the subject of decades of heated debate, with so-called "Lyme-literate doctors" and chronic patients on one side fighting a pitched battle against the medical establishment, exemplified by the Infectious Disease Society of America, over the underlying cause and therefore treatment of chronic symptoms in some Lyme patients.

Lyme-literate doctors argue that patients' ongoing symptoms may be driven by the *B. burgdorferi* bacterium, or other tick-borne infections, stealthily persisting in the body's tissues, evading the body's immune response. If so, then the infection can be eradicated by long-term courses of antibiotics, not unlike the plan my doctor prescribed. However, most academic specialists argue that there isn't evidence of the bacteria persisting in the human body after the standard course of a few weeks of antibiotics, and many doubt whether chronic Lyme is a real disease at all. Regimens of antibiotics for months or years could do more harm than good, the IDSA argues. And a handful of placebo-controlled clinical trials haven't borne substantive evidence that long-term antibiotics are appropriate.

Given the controversy of this disease, patients with post-treatment Lyme disease syndrome are often left desperately fumbling through a medical underground of contested science and alternative practitioners. Unproven or even bizarre treatments become vastly preferable to a mainstream that tells them their disabling symptoms are psychosomatic, and don't have a basis in objective fact.

Lyme is part of a class of "great imitators," a designation given to diseases with wide-ranging or non-specific symptoms that overlap with other diseases. For great imitators, which can include fibromyalgia, multiple sclerosis, and lupus, there's a high chance for misdiagnosis. Just as in Covid long haulers, Lyme can begin with an acute infection that apparently resolves, but then later produces long-term fatigue, pain, and cognitive dysfunction even though patients appear to come up normal on routine lab tests.

The symptom presentation in post-treatment Lyme disease syndrome and Long Covid patients is "remarkably similar," said Dr. John Aucott, director of the Johns Hopkins University Lyme Disease Research Center. He was amazed at early studies of Long Covid patients with bar graphs showing the prevalence of major symptoms. If you placed those charts alongside self-reported symptoms of Lyme "long haulers," it was almost like they were mirror images of each other.

That suggested to him perhaps the best corollary to Long Covid came from previous insights in ME/CFS and POTS, disorders marked by decreased blood flow to the brain, and associated with inflammation in the autonomic nervous system, the part of the nervous system that directs automatic functions of the body. The autonomic nervous system tells the heart to beat at seventy beats per minute while sitting at rest or the lungs to breathe faster while running sprints—tasks that don't require active thinking. So even though organs themselves weren't damaged in Lyme or Long Covid, the heart or lungs or GI tract didn't work properly because the part of the nervous system that controlled them was affected.

One way that autonomic nervous system disruption could be explained is by altered function of your vagus nerve, Aucott explained to me over the phone one afternoon in the fall of 2021. "Maybe you're not getting enough blood to your brain because of altered autonomic control of your blood pressure and pulse, which is triggered when the vagus nerve is inflamed or triggered by the infection," Aucott said.

"That's one hypothesis that ties it all together," he said. "It seems to explain why all the symptoms look the same in chronic fatigue and long haul Covid and Lyme, because maybe they all share that same mechanism. They're seeing tons of autonomic dysfunction in long haul Covid."

And few doctors fully understand the underlying mechanics because there's limited teaching about autonomic nervous system disorders in medical school.

There are plenty of other hypotheses to explore for why Lyme triggers long-term illness. But progress in studying the profoundly life-altering condition has plodded along with poor funding. To be sure, NIH funding levels have slowly ticked upward from $20 million in 2013 to an estimated $50 million in 2021. So far though, there haven't been enough resources to get a solid handle on the different possible underlying mechanisms of the illness. But even though mainstream medicine couldn't agree on the exact nature of the fire, the smoke looks very similar to Long Covid.

"From Lyme disease, I think the lesson may be more that infection can trigger persistent inflammation. That is the potential mechanism for why the patient doesn't get better," Aucott said. "To what extent post-treatment Lyme is just classic autoimmunity versus just persistent inflammation, that's still not clear."

Another lesson from Lyme could come in evidence that the pieces of the *B. burgdorferi* bacteria could be triggering long-term illness, just as fragments of SARS-CoV-2 might be doing the same for Covid patients.

"There actually is some intriguing data in Lyme disease that the proteins that make up the cell walls of the bacteria may linger in the tissues, and perpetuate inflammation," Aucott told me. "Even after the viable organisms are gone and dead. But there are pieces or bits of protein that are lying around triggering ongoing inflammation." During fifteen years of research, Aucott and his research team at Johns Hopkins have published studies showing a range of ways that Lyme appeared to cause persistent inflammation, rewiring neural networks in a way that became self-perpetuating even if the original infection truly had been eradicated.

The team had found elevated levels of a cytokine called CCL19, which stood out among dozens of inflammatory markers in long-term Lyme. They also found that gene regulation patterns are highly abnormal in post-treatment Lyme disease syndrome patients. In essence, while doctors would expect that genes regulating an immune response would be active for a few weeks during the acute phase of an infection, Aucott's team showed they were significantly altered six months after infection. That helped build a picture similar to other Lyme studies of the metabolome—the full spectrum of metabolites and other small molecules in the body—showing that the metabolic processes were altered for long periods of time and didn't return to normal after they were treated.

Similar to Covid, if the original pathogen was no longer detectable—at least through conventional means—then doctors were left to treat the symptoms, working with patients to manage their sleep, pain, and fatigue issues with existing drugs even though they couldn't solve the underlying problem outright. Proving definitively whether human Lyme infections could persist or enter the brain was difficult partially due to the few available autopsy studies on subjects with Lyme. Researchers can get ethics approval to poke around the brains of infected mice that they've sacrificed ahead of time. Since Lyme is rarely deadly, there was limited opportunity to repeat the same studies in humans. However, even if Lyme doesn't kill people directly, plenty of people with Lyme die from other causes, so these types of studies could be done by setting up established biobanks for human biopsy and autopsy tissues from Lyme disease patients.

"There is some evidence in animal models for sequestered hidden infections where the bacteria—even after antibiotics—may be hiding in a kind of dormant state in privileged sites in which the immune system can't get rid of them," Aucott said.

A similar problem presented in Covid, due to ethical and practical difficulties of performing brain autopsy studies in human subjects. Early autopsy studies by the NIH hadn't found SARS-CoV-2 in the brain, although a German study of patients who had died of Covid suggested otherwise, finding viral proteins in isolated cells in the brainstem. It was an early clue there could at least be a possibility that Covid brain fog was driven by virus infiltrating part of the brain. It wouldn't be until December 2021 that scientists from the NIH released preprint results, prior to peer review, of a more robust autopsy study that definitively found persistent SARS-CoV-2 in the brain and throughout the body.

One of the best ways around those issues is through the increased use of more sophisticated brain imaging techniques in recent years, offering a chance to "dissect" the brain of a living creature without physically cutting into it.

In a 2018 neuroimaging study, Aucott's group had demonstrated neuroinflammation from Lyme using positron emission tomography (PET) scans, the same type of imaging used to show proof of brain damage in living former NFL players. In that study, they found post-treatment Lyme patients had activated glial cells, a type of immune cell in the central nervous system. That type of PET scan isn't readily accessible for practicing physicians, but they point to a real underlying biology for the hellish aftermath of Lyme.

Beyond new technologies, the pandemic might be forcing a cultural shift, exposing whole new swaths of the health profession and society at large to rethink post-infectious, or para-infectious diseases, bringing them into the light.

"Covid is actually exciting because it's gotten people's attention on this at a much bigger scale. I think that's helpful for us," he said. "It's not as easy to deny Long Covid because of the scale of the issue."

Those similarities prompted researchers from Stanford University to adapt another set of new technologies to design a way to see into the daily lives of patients. In October 2021, they launched a two-year "Crash Course" study comparing people with ME/CFS, Lyme, and Long Covid to learn how and why they all experience the trademark post-exertional crashes common in each condition. These dynamic "continuous sensing" side-by-side comparisons of all three diseases might reveal common characteristics across each of them. The researchers gave each participant a wearable Fitbit device to keep track of daily heart rate, step count, sleep, and other variables. Each participant would collect sixteen blood samples over the course of a three-month period using an innovative at-home blood draw device called a Tasso. Some would be baseline measures, and others would specifically show how they felt on a good day versus on a crash day.

Chapter 13

THEORY OF EVERYTHING

For more than a century, physicists have been feverishly searching for what scientists call the "Theory of Everything." A theory so flexible and all-encompassing that it would unite all the laws of the universe. Albert Einstein contributed a huge piece of the puzzle when he first described the phenomenon of general relativity, the rules that governed large scale physics like space, time, and gravity. Around the same time, another concept was emerging known as quantum mechanics, which is the study of very, *very* small matter, like atoms and their sub-particles, and the laws that they abide by. With these two grand theories, both big and small, it may come as a surprise that the puzzle of "everything" did not fit together. Quantum mechanics and the theory of relativity are ultimately incompatible. The rules of one did not hold up when applied to the other. What huge puzzle piece were physicists missing? Despite the genius of the subsequent generations, physicists have not yet been able to synthesize the laws of physics into an overall single theory to explain them all. And yet we know that some explainable order of the cosmos has to exist.

The field of human biology is a tricky science to design perfectly repeatable experiments around, as it usually proves hard to control the plethora of confounding variables. However, when it comes to disease, the need for a Theory of Everything is just as urgent as in the cosmos and the particles. Study after study has shown us an abundance of abnormalities across many systems in diseases like ME/CFS, Long Covid, and Lyme. Some researchers have been looking at the smaller cellular level examining mitochondria, blood vessels and endothelial cells, natural killer cells, and cytokine disruptions. At the same time, other researchers have taken a more biological systems approach and focused on characteristics of the gut microbiome, connective tissue, autonomic dysfunction, the vagus nerve, mechanical instabilities, and the brainstem. And in an arguably even more global approach to the body, some scientists focus squarely on patient symptoms like post-exertional malaise and cognitive issues to guide their research into post-viral illness. But it seems just when we have our hands around the castle, it turns to sand. Is it possible, just as in physics, as we look at the same problem from different angles or maybe even more importantly *at different time points*, that the problem shape shifts, evading a unifying theory?

"Unless we follow these things from the beginning, we won't be able to tie those things together. There's lots of information that we're already starting to see in Long Covid. It's a post-viral syndrome, it's got all these immune abnormalities," said Dr. Lucinda Bateman, the Chief Medical Officer at the Bateman Horne Center of Excellence in Salt Lake City, Utah . "There's a lot of neurological symptoms. There's actually quite a bit of mitochondrial dysfunction as well. It'll be interesting to see if the story of Long Covid pulls all those together to see how they relate to each other."

Maybe Covid is our Big Bang. We have to start at the beginning.

Is it also possible that most accepted and well-described diseases behave according to a theory of everything but are not subject to this level of scrutiny and doubt from the medical community and society at large? Perhaps it's because most of these conditions have a definable and agreed upon biomarker that is readily testable. For example, if you have a pattern of specific lesions in the brain, you may be diagnosed with multiple sclerosis. However, when you look at the biology of patients with MS, it is clearly a complex disease, with abundant red flags across multiple systems. Without the biomarker, MS might just be as confusing as ME/CFS seems now.

For now, the primary physical reaction to an infectious agent like Covid or Lyme that eventually sets off the chain of events that often leads to a new stubborn homeostasis of disease is stumping the scientific community. Maybe the infection hits multiple systems at once. In fact, is it preposterous to zoom farther out and assume all diseased states within the body are long-standing effects of assaults from viruses, bacteria, vaccines, parasites, and the like? In cases like multiple sclerosis or Alzheimer's, we don't know yet who walked in that room and flipped that switch, though some hypothesize it might've been a virus. At least in these diseases, however, we know quite a bit more about which switch it was. Sometimes we know the switch *and* who flipped it, like with HIV/AIDS.

What is clear is that at some point, the infection-associated diseases such as Long Covid and ME/CFS look like a circular merry-go-round from hell, with no way to know what came first or what is perpetuating what between vagus nerve damage, leaky blood vessels, connective tissue fragility, etc. And worst of all, it's not clear how to get off the ride. And maybe by the time you have had it for long enough, it doesn't matter what came first. You're stuck. A growing body of research points to some sort of switch getting flipped, throwing people into a long-term state of illness. Interestingly, in the case of Long Covid, we know *who* flipped the switch: it was SARS-CoV-2.

"One of the problems is that it's a hypometabolic state," Ron Davis, professor of genetics at Stanford University, told me during a wide-ranging conversation about the many avenues of dysfunction in the disease and the quest to neatly sum them all up. In a hypometabolic state, the body's metabolic processes are suppressed and normal activities are suspended.

"For ME/CFS there's a lot of metabolites that are very low level, probably because the mitochondria have been partially shut down," he said. "We're looking at some of the pathways in mitochondria in great detail. Mitochondria are clearly involved in this in some way and that needs to get explored."

THE PUZZLE SOLVER

It's been nine years since I first searched the name "Ron Davis" in a Stanford dorm room before interviewing him in 2013, and I learned about his career earning dozens of patents as a pioneer of the technology that drove the Human Genome Project. At the time, he had just dropped his entire research agenda to focus on ME/CFS after his son developed a severe case of the disease, becoming bedridden for a decade and unable to eat or swallow solid food. Davis vowed that for as long as he lived, he would fight on behalf of his son and the millions around the world with the same disease.

Over the past decade, he injected new vigor and rigor into the field, recruiting new researchers with a pitch that ME/CFS is the "last great disease left to conquer." He joined a National Academy of Medicine committee convened by the federal government, which reviewed the full body of thousands of peer-reviewed research studies. It published the 2015 report that suggested a new name for the illness, "systemic exertion intolerance disease," based around its foremost clinical sign. It was the consolidation of everything known to date about ME/CFS, and called for a new way forward for research, clinical care, and medical education, recommending dramatic increases across each area. Davis built a network of dozens of scientists and several collaborative research centers around the world, including at Stanford, Harvard, and Uppsala University in Sweden. The Open Medicine Foundation, where he is the lead scientific advisor, raised more than $30 million for research.

All the while, Davis and his wife, Janet Dafoe, arranged each aspect of their daily lives toward responding to their son's needs. Multiple times each day, they sat outside Whitney's room, head bowed, waiting for their son's signal that it's all right to come inside his room. They hook up IV drips for hydration, wash his feet, and clip his toenails. For years, they wore plain shirts without lettering because even the sliver of energy it takes for Whitney to process a word could cause him to crash, triggering severe stomach pain that made it impossible to put more food into his feeding tube. Caring for Whitney, monitoring his every bodily signal, was one of Davis' central ways of generating new ideas to test out and new drugs to try. With a port in his chest, Whitney was an easy source of blood draws, and often served as an initial guinea pig for studies. Whitney had the starkest form of ME/CFS, and cases like his might serve as a benchmark for the trajectory in which the illness could progress in some cases. The OMF funded a study of severe ME/CFS, believing that whatever was wrong at a fundamental level would be most clear or apparent for those with the direst cases. Whitney's symptoms represented the most extreme reality for sufferers of post-viral illness, like Long Covid. Where the disease is paints the body in its boldest and most destructive colors, its individual brushstrokes might be most discernible.

And those brushstrokes, Davis believes, are most likely rooted at the molecular level. He and his team designed an ultrasensitive "nanoneedle" device that could test for that molecular signature from a single drop of blood. In 2019, they published initial findings in the journal Proceedings of the National Academy of Sciences showing that in a study of forty patients and healthy control subjects that their nanoneedle could distinguish each time whether the person had the illness or not. Patients' blood responded to a stressor—in this case, salt.

"What we don't know is whether other diseases show the same thing," Davis said. "And it doesn't prove anything until we can do a number of other infections."

Getting the nanoneedle to work at scale might mean a biomarker for the disease and could eventually lead to creating a blood test to diagnose the condition quickly and easily. From there, they could compare the marker to a catalog of drugs already approved by the FDA which could be repurposed to treat ME/CFS.

As the beginning of the pandemic took shape, Davis saw another opportunity to deploy advanced techniques such as systems biology, genome sequencing, and metabolomics to observe the likely beginnings of the ME/CFS and try to learn if and how a switch gets flipped, transitioning the person into a chronic illness. They enrolled Covid-19 patients in a new study so they could collect regular samples over a period of years and monitor which people developed a longer-term post-viral fatigue syndrome. Having data on patients from the beginning of an illness like Covid and observing them longitudinally over time as the illness progresses gives Davis and his team a unique opportunity to capture the disease process and increases the likelihood of discovering the molecular Holy Grail.

Davis had prominence, a prestigious collaborative network, and significant headway into understanding post-viral conditions. As expert patient leaders living with Long Covid began meeting with planners of the NIH's big initiative to study long haulers, Ron Davis's research agenda—and of a dozen others established in the field—appeared to be obvious and relevant to their ongoing plight. At the same time, a different Davis, the Patient-Led Research Collaborative's Hannah Davis, was so worried that RECOVER Initiative planners might not take prior post-viral research into consideration with Long Covid that she gave them a presentation in the summer of 2021 highlighting more than a dozen current clinicians and scientists who had spent their careers working on these complex syndromes, who might have the most relevant experience and most promising leads within a field that conventional medicine had consistently bobbled for decades. She highlighted their ongoing lines of research: Michael VanElzakker and his work in neuroinflammation, Nancy Klimas and her career in post-infectious immunology, and Avindra Nath and his ongoing intramural study within the NIH itself.

Hannah Davis included Ron Davis among those high on the list that she and patients hoped would be included in the RECOVER Initiative. The PLRC leader thought his team's nanoneedle technology might provide the basis for eventually discerning a biomarker in the blood for Long Covid.

The genome pioneer felt the same way, linking ME/CFS and Long Covid.

"I'd be surprised if they're actually different," Ron Davis said. Symptomatically, the basic differences between ME/CFS and Long Covid disappear in the months after the acute infection. "They're different in one way, in that ME/CFS was ignored and Long Covid was not."

His team applied for two grants to study Long Covid, but both were rejected on the grounds that he was collecting molecular data. Other longtime post-viral researchers whom the patients recommended didn't make the cut either, for one reason or another. He was in fundamental disagreement with the pieces of feedback he received in his rejection.

"One of them specifically said that I couldn't run any of the data, I had to archive it. I would have to collect blood samples, and then freeze them, but not study them," Davis said. The initiative intended to set up a biorepository of samples so that many teams of researchers could study them for their different projects.

For him, those kinds of logistical considerations were a huge problem in designing the careful experiments required to tease out the source of the disease. The Stanford Genome Technology Center's nanoneedle device—which might hold the key to discovering a biomarker for ME/CFS and therefore Long Covid—didn't work on frozen blood samples. "We've tried and tried and tried to find a way that preserves them, but we haven't found that. Just that fact alone says that changes are occurring in the blood when you freeze it. We don't know what is changing but we know something is changing. And that could be key to what's actually happening in the immune system and cause people to miss it."

The Open Medicine Foundation found an initial $1 million in funding at the beginning of the pandemic to study post-Covid patients, starting with post-ICU patients they had access to through their center in Sweden. While they had a small amount of private money available to study long haulers, the bulk of the organization's funding came from private donations earmarked for ME/CFS. Running their tests on both sets of patient communities in comparison groups side-by-side was almost assured to garner the most useful results but wouldn't be fair to the patients who'd originally donated to study their own disease.

"I am very resistant to taking donation money from patients that suffer with ME/CFS to study Long Covid. It just seems unethical to me," he told me. "There's lots of money for Long Covid, hundreds of times more money than for ME/CFS. And why should the ME/CFS patients pay for trying to understand Long Covid?"

Such is the dilemma of siloes. The private scraps available for one disease were in one pot, and the large public outlays for its nearly identical twin were in a different pot out of reach.

Davis and his team are working to prove or disprove whether patients' cells enter a "metabolic trap" that disrupts the molecular process for energy production. The science is a complicated two-step involving a pair of genes. The first gene, IDO1, works to process the amino acid tryptophan into compounds involved in regulating the immune system, reducing inflammation in the brain, and producing the energy molecule ATP. If there's too much tryptophan in a cell, IDO1 can get overwhelmed and can't produce the compounds that underpin healthy immune functioning and energy production. A major insult to the body, such as a viral infection, can increase tryptophan and overload IDO1. There's a backup gene, IDO2, ensuring the body keeps producing energy as normal. But 65 percent of the human population has a mutation there. That's not a problem if the first system never gets overwhelmed, but if exposed to a powerful virus such as SARS-CoV-2, it could be enough to flip the switch.

"One way to study this is that we would like to put a cell into a trap, which we can do in yeast and human immune cells to see how to get the cell out of a trap with a drug," he told me. "We have completed our screening of all the FDA-approved drugs for yeast. We have a number of compounds that will get yeast out of the trap."

If the metabolic trap is proven, it might be a keystone helping hold together the myriad of symptoms and far-flung clinical observations in the disease.

Davis didn't want to get too excited about certain Long Covid drugs that generated a certain amount of early buzz. For a desperate patient community, directing too much hope to a hot new treatment too early can lead to disappointments, especially when they might only work well for a small subset of patients or if the positive effects proved fleeting. New findings garner headlines and generate glimmers of hope in patient communities. However, the research process is slow and may or may not bear the kind of fruit that ultimately results in drugs reaching the finish line for FDA approval. Beyond that, many new drugs and interventions can be overly expensive or lack a financial model by which the treatment can be distributed widely and equitably. The ideal solution would be repurposing a drug already on pharmacy shelves, rather than bringing a brand new compound to market, a process often cited as requiring about a decade and at least $1 billion to complete. In order to reach the greatest number of people, research findings would have to be reproducible across multiple trials, and treatments would ideally be fairly inexpensive.

Berlin Cures, a pharmaceutical company in Germany, generated fanfare by successfully treating several patients in the summer of 2021 with a new compound called BC 007, which was originally developed to treat heart disease. Administered in a little over an hour by IV drip, the drug acts to improve blood flow and may reduce autoantibodies circulating in the body long after Covid infection. By early 2022, the company was enrolling dozens more patients in a clinical trial. Davis was keen to collaborate with them.

"I don't know if it's going to be a cure or not. But it could be a treatment, which could be great," Davis said.

But he warned that the trail of clinical research is often littered with disappointments, so keeping a judicious eye on the big picture mattered. Many long haulers get thrown into the murky backwaters of experimental treatments, desperately seeking anything that might get their lives back beyond just trying to manage their symptoms.

PUZZLE PIECES IN LONG COVID RESEARCH

Pieces of the puzzle continue to emerge, with a stream of studies confirming the persistence of SARS-CoV-2 in the body along with inflammation, autoantibody activity, and deterioration of the endothelial cells that line blood vessels.

So far, there's no simple equation or theory of everything to describe the underlying disease, and there's no simple protocol to follow in treating it. But it hasn't stopped brilliantly determined investigators like Amy Proal, a microbiologist at the PolyBio Research Foundation, from trying. The perpetually crumbling sandcastle is beginning to congeal.

As mentioned in chapter eight, Proal worked with her colleague Mike VanElzakker to review the research from the first two years of the pandemic—as well as the history of science focused on infection-associated chronic diseases. She neatly folded them into a unified framework for thinking about Long Covid. She sees seven major factors driving cycles within the body that lead into the persisting illness, which provide the basis for the many teams of researchers working to understand, treat, and eventually cure the disease.

First, at least some of the long-term disease in Long Covid can be directly attributed to a measurable organ injury such as lung, heart, or kidney damage. But a standard echocardiogram or blood test can usually see that right away. From there, though, things get much more interesting.

The vast majority of patients may have a set of underlying pathologies that require robust judgment and attention from doctors to discern. Additionally, the field needs innovation in diagnostics so that the most relevant abnormalities could stand out. According to Proal's analysis of the ongoing research in the field, Long Covid manifests as a combination of some or all of the following: persistence of the SARS-CoV-2 virus, reactivation of other persistent pathogens, dysregulation of the patient's microbiome or virome, blood coagulation, extended autoantibody production, and disruption of vagus nerve signaling to the brainstem. Because the disease is heterogenous, the exact version of those factors would manifest differently depending on the myriad of complexities of a particular body.

Your average nasal swab or blood test won't pick up on persistent virus after the acute stage of the infection is over, a fact that has complicated the understanding of lingering viral loads. Rather, residual virus can hide out in tissues. Studies have increasingly shown that SARS-CoV-2 is *capable of persistence*. Researchers from the NIH performed forty-four autopsies. All had been infected with SARS-CoV-2. Some had been asymptomatic while others had died from Covid. The results, posted as a preprint in December 2021 ahead of a publication in the journal *Nature*, offered definitive evidence that the virus could dwell in the brain. In early January 2022, it was top of mind for Dr. Anthony Fauci when Sen. Tim Kaine—who regularly made a point to ask about Long Covid—posed a query to the expert about the NIH's progress helping long haulers during a Senate health committee hearing. He explained that an individual could test negative for the virus via nasal swab while the virus persisted in anatomical sanctuaries throughout the body, including the cardiovascular, gastrointestinal, renal, endocrine, and reproductive tissues. In one case they found the virus lasting in tissues for up to 230 days, the full length of the study. The autopsies showed that the virus could likely enter the brain by crossing the blood-brain barrier, and lodge itself in the brainstem. It was the most high-quality study to that point proving widespread SARS-CoV-2 viral reservoirs.

The next puzzle piece—*reactivation of persistent pathogens*—highlights how some of the dysfunction in post-infectious illness stems from older pathogens in the body that are newly emboldened to cause damage again. "Under conditions of health these viruses are kept in check by the immune system," Proal says. "The immune system has defenses that keep them in a largely dormant or inactive state. But, and this is a well-known phenomenon under conditions of stress, the same viruses can reactivate and begin to drive symptoms." Most humans accumulate a range of viruses throughout their lifetimes, including multiple strains of herpesviruses. Many people with Long Covid experience reactivations of latent herpesviruses, which can manifest in cold sores or as shingles. That phenomenon, long established in the literature of chronic illnesses, isn't new in Long Covid. In one study of Long Covid patients, some two-thirds showed Epstein-Barr virus reactivation, compared with just 10 percent of controls.

The human body contains trillions of organisms, the sum total of which make up what's called the microbiome. Another area of Long Covid is *dysregulation of host microbiome*, Proal explains. Similar to how Covid-19 leads to virus reactivation, it can also tip the balance in the microbiome, shifting the homeostasis characterizing normal function.

Those phenomena together help lead into the category of *endothelial cell damage, platelet hyperactivation, and blood coagulation.* While it is clear these mechanisms are implicated in symptomatology during acute Covid infection, researchers are finding persistent dysfunction across these areas in Long Covid patients as well. These anomalies could help link multiple factors together. Each reactivation of virus and bacteria can cause inflammation and sometimes direct infection of endothelial cells, the cells lining the blood vessels. As platelets in the blood—which contribute to the dysfunction in more ways than one—react to these microvascular injuries, they clump together into microclots. If the blood becomes clotted because of Long Covid, it makes it harder for oxygen and nutrient-rich components to perfuse tissue throughout the body, and that can contribute to small fiber neuropathy, a kind of nerve damage. The clots could be a major contributor to the post-exertional malaise most long haulers feel. In addition, as endothelial cells maintain the integrity of tissue barriers and also mediate both innate and acquired immunity, injuries to these cells can cause increased permeability in the membranes throughout the body, including those in the gut and the brain. Even here, you can start to get an appreciation of the snowball rolling down the hill, gathering weight, mass, and speed as each assault builds on the previous one and sets the stage for a new dysfunction.

In a study, Harvard's Dr. David Systrom used a process called invasive cardiopulmonary testing to find abnormal blood flow throughout the body, including blood flowing to the brain. In that test, researchers insert a catheter into a subject's vein with a tiny balloon in it that can take measurements of factors in their blood while they ride an exercise bike. They brought ten people with Long Covid into their process used for studying exercise intolerance in ME/CFS and a range of diseases. Sure enough, they found that each of the ten long haulers demonstrated impaired oxygen extraction. And the reduced blood flow to the brain could be a primary driver of the brain fog so many patients report.

Notably, of the four types of tissue in the body—connective, epithelial, muscle, and nervous—connective tissue is of particular interest to some researchers. Connective tissue, a cohesive structural tissue that supports organs and other bodily tissues and includes cartilage, fat, bone, blood, and connective tissue proper, has been implicated in a number of post-pathogen disease states. Proal added, "it would be strange if connective tissue would be sterile." As mentioned above, blood, a type of connective tissue, is significantly affected by Covid-19. It's possible the virus degrades other connective tissue as well. After all, Proal states, a pathogen like "*Borrelia burgdorferi*—the bacterium found in Lyme disease—is a known connective tissue degrader." There are many diseases and disorders of connective tissue, such as Ehlers-Danlos syndrome. Some are genetic, while others are acquired, or epigenetic, coming from an interaction between genes and the environment.

There is an abundance of ways diseases of connective tissue can show up, and many look very different from each other. One common outcome is when connective tissue fails to provide adequate support in ligaments, joints, and skin. The results can be a plethora of structural instabilities that cause painful and disabling neurological symptoms, many of which have been noted in patient accounts of those suffering from ME/CFS and POTS. These instabilities are caused by weakened structural connective tissue. For instance, craniocervical instability, or CCI, is associated with diminished connective tissue around the craniocervical area that holds the head and spine in proper position. Weak ligamentous connections around the base of the skull or in other spinal regions can lead to pressure or stretching as internal elements compress or stretch important anatomy including the spinal cord and deep brain areas, including the vagus nerve. The resulting symptoms become disabling and serve as one more example of the myriad ways in which a particular syndrome has a web of possible underlying causes. In the case of CCI, a surgery might repair the underlying problem and set the patient back toward good health.

Finally, Proal's model relies on *disruption of vagus nerve signaling*. The widely branching nerve has major receptors that innervate every major organ in the body, and a disruption of the vagus nerve was proposed by Michael VanElzakker as a major explanation for ME/CFS in 2013. It's also a direct highway to the dorsal brainstem. Under ideal conditions, the vagus nerve can maintain immune homeostasis and regulate autonomic and metabolic function. Under conditions of possible persistent infection, like those seen in Long Covid, the balance is upset. If there is a SARS-CoV-2 reservoir, a reactivated virus, a disrupted microbiome, or structural compression, then the vagus nerve can sense inflammation and send a signal to the brainstem, triggering neural cells that cause what's known as a "sickness response." And it's not just a signal and a subjective feeling of illness, the vagus nerve can elicit neuroinflammation, disrupting vital signals throughout the brain. VanElzakker's PET scan studies in ME/CFS have shown a kind of brain inflammation that likely contributed to brain fog and are now being rolled out in Long Covid. Proal points out, "no one gets this sick without the brain involved."

The model distills many areas of complex and emerging science into a set of themes, which can vary person to person. Long

Covid probably isn't one-size-fits-all. Any particular patient might have any individualized version of the mix of factors that Proal outlines.

Proal ran through a few different scenarios depicting how the various factors could play out in a particular individual. In one scenario, the SARS-CoV-2 virus could have formed a reservoir in a person's intestines, resulting in inflammation that triggers the vagus nerve to send a proinflammatory signal to the dorsal brainstem that resulted in the person feeling sickness, pain, nausea, and autonomic symptoms. Simultaneously, proteins from the virus could leak into the blood, leading to distortions in coagulation and the vasculature as well as low oxygen levels in tissue.

In another scenario, a patient might have totally cleared SARS-CoV-2 from every part of the body. But then the Epstein-Barr virus, lying dormant up to that point, could have seized on the opportunity of a temporarily weakened immune system to reactivate. In Proal's example, this patient also has significant gut dysbiosis, in which the diverse microbial ecosystem in the GI is disordered. The patient's Epstein-Barr reactivation and gut issues then trigger a similar proinflammatory signal up through the vagus nerve and the dorsal brainstem set off the same feelings of sickness, pain, nausea, and autonomic symptoms. This person could also be a Covid long hauler, with the virus setting off a chain of events even after leaving the body. Rather than persistent infection, this person might be the victim of a hit-and-run.

Still, a third person might have similar symptoms, but a third set of underlying factors to their Long Covid. In this storyline, SARS-CoV-2 sets up shop long-term in lung tissue in a person who might already have had an enterovirus infection in the stomach and oral microbiome dysbiosis. This person, with Covid-19 being just one of multiple hits to their system, becomes even sicker through the same process of the vagus nerve signaling a three-alarm fire of systemic sickness response throughout the body.

The examples could go on and on, of course, substituting different underlying infections, different host sites for SARS-CoV-2, and different routes of disruption.

MOVING FORWARD BY LOOKING INTO THE PAST

Proal's own life experience of nearly dying from microbial infection would inspire a lifetime researching the roots and triggers of chronic illness. She grew up in Mexico City, and as a young girl she was hospitalized for a series of measles, rubella, scarlet fever, and pneumonia infections. She barely survived. Her slew of encephalitic infections appeared to quiet down, and she grew into a successful high school athlete, later captaining the school's tennis team. While an undergraduate at Georgetown University, though, some sort of illness began to plague her. The illness left her bedridden for eight months, unable to tolerate light or sound. Doctors at the school's health center couldn't figure it out, and she barely pulled off graduating.

"I just started, when I could, to read about infections and slowly, slowly try to understand if any of the infections that I'd had might have contributed to my case because I didn't know what could have happened," Proal said.

She began reaching out to longstanding researchers studying infections and launched into a series of experimental treatments supporting her immune system along with pulse antibiotics to wear down bacterial infection and "a huge number of antivirals." She got herself back up and functioning and was eventually the lead author of a paper in *Immunologic Research* on immuno-stimulation in the treatment of ME/CFS. That experience propelled her to pursue her PhD in microbiology and polish the lens through which she observed the infectious roots of complex illness.

She formed the PolyBio Research Foundation with Harvard neuroscientist Michael VanElzakker, who had a close friend with a similar story to Proal's. Their constant observation of symptoms—of close friends and those in patient networks—helps them generate new hypotheses. "One of these things that both Mike and I do is we actually just listen and talk to the patients that we know in our lives and on Twitter. That's a huge part of how we come up with what we're going to study."

In 2019, *before* the pandemic, Proal reached out to South African scientist Resia Pretorius, a leader in the field of blood clotting who had conducted research into how clotting was connected to diabetes and related conditions. Proal was impressed by Pretorius' work showing how platelets activated in response to bacteria and viruses. So, she wanted to study how proteins from enteroviruses and herpesviruses activated platelets and contributed to clotting in ME/CFS patients' blood.

"While we were working to get that off the ground, Covid started. So Resia's team started to look at clotting in acute Covid and Long Covid, and I just jumped in pretty quickly," she said. "Ironically, that Long Covid data was out before the ME/CFS data, but they just started to find *clear* microclots in the blood of basically every Long Covid subject analyzed, which is pretty rare, and puts them in the mind of some researchers as potentially the first bio-marker for Long Covid."

Pretorius and her team found the microclots by looking at long haulers' blood under a fluorescence microscope, using techniques not widely available in conventional medical settings.

Under normal circumstances, blood should form clots if you cut your finger. The clots would soon break up via a process called fibrinolysis. But in many Long Covid patients, they found, the tiny clots didn't break up, and inflammatory molecules were trapped inside them, where they could avoid detection in routine blood tests that made deeply distressed patients come up looking healthy. The molecules that help break down clots were stuck inside the clots themselves.

"A regular doctor or clinical center is not going to be able to see the clots, so you have to go through a series of steps to make them show up in your sample. They published that in their paper, so teams can replicate that now," Proal explained.

The next step involved training other research teams to find the clots in a variety of different ways, for instance using the lab technique called flow cytometry, which filters the blood down and measures characteristics of the sample, and some groups showed success in detecting the clots that way in addition to microscopy.

"If you know how to find them, it's not very hard," Proal told me. "So it's not a dream that you could go to a Long Covid clinical care center and that they could have a little lab where they could look for the clots."

The sticky blood has more trouble flowing throughout the body. The South African researchers found a strong signal in those with post-Covid symptoms who improved after a month of treatment with a protocol that included antiplatelet and anticoagulant drugs, as well as proton pump inhibitor. That also led the team toward looking into apheresis treatments, a process similar to dialysis, which clears out harmful molecules from the blood. The apheresis process is expensive and would require continual visits to a clinic with the right equipment for patients to continue experiencing positive effects, but if the initial case studies lead to positive results in randomized control trials, it could become a more mainstream option.

But it's not just the here and now Proal and researchers like her worry about. The brain damage in long haulers could lead to dramatic increases in dementia, Alzheimer's, and Parkinson's, fitting an emergent consensus about the infectious roots of many brain diseases. "The idea that the brain is sterile and that it's not infected is falling. It's just crumbling," Proal said. Now that we know SARS-CoV-2 infects the brain directly and is persistent in tissues long after the acute illness is over, this fact opens the door to other questions about what happens to infection in the brain long term.

What was once a fringe theory that viruses might contribute to devastating neurodegenerative diseases like Alzheimer's is now gaining mainstream traction. In 2018, scientist Leslie Norins offered $1 million to any scientist who could demonstrate that Alzheimer's disease was caused by a germ. "There's all kinds of connections between existing virus and neurodegenerative disease," Proal said. After all, no one believed *Heliobacter pylori* triggered stomach ulcers and many could not have guessed that Epstein-Barr virus was a precursor for multiple sclerosis, two facts we now accept. In the case of Alzheimer's disease, which accounts for 60 to 70 percent of all dementia, the "amyloid beta hypothesis," which postulates that toxic plaques consisting of amyloid beta protein and noxious tangles of tau proteins damage neurons and cause widespread brain inflammation, accounting for the devastating symptoms. While there was generally a consensus around this hypothesis for years, the field has stumbled in its efforts to break apart the plaques and tangles in a manner that significantly relieves symptoms of the disease, leaving the cohort of researchers scratching their heads.

As interest in what's known as the "infection theory" has grown, many researchers are beginning to understand that the two theories are not mutually exclusive. "Overall, amyloid beta seems to act as part of the innate immune response toward infection in brain tissue and is highly conserved, which usually means it's been selected for and it's continued to occur because it has a function," says Proal. One group of experiments led by Ruth Itzhaki, now an emeritus professor at the University of Manchester in the UK, in the 1990s hypothesized that repeated reactivation of a herpesvirus, HSV-1, was causing the buildup of amyloid plaques in patient's brains. The researchers found that the viral infection *and* the presence of the APOE4 gene variant led to a significant increase in Alzheimer's risk. One without the other: not so much. Although originally met with suspicion, this finding has been replicated many times over.

Although no single lab won the $1 million reward for identifying the sole microbe implicated in causing Alzheimer's disease, Itzhaki's group split the prize with seven other researchers who identified six different infectious agents in the brains of Alzheimer's patients. With six different microbes identified in the brains of these subjects, it's possible multiple agents can cause what we refer to as Alzheimer's disease. If this is the case, Alzheimer's might come to be known as an "umbrella" term, indicating an infection in the brain. Much like pneumonia or diarrhea, the condition might be treatable in its symptomology as well as at its infectious origin. Interestingly, a large study in 2018 showed that treatment with antivirals was associated with a reduced risk of dementia in those carrying the herpes simplex virus. Other studies have found that a herpes zoster infection (also known as shingles) is associated with increased risk of dementia, and that the bacterium associated with gum disease, *Porphyromonas gingivalis*, may trigger the accumulation of amyloid beta. Coronaviruses, including SARS-CoV-2, are neurotropic, meaning they are capable on infecting the nervous system. So is not a far stretch then to wonder if SARS-CoV-2 could predispose a population of survivors to increased dementia risk. "Why wouldn't SARS coronavirus be one of those viruses?" Proal pondered. The tide is undoubtedly turning, at least in scientific circles. An international consortium, made up of the Alzheimer's Association and representatives from more than twenty-five countries, are exploring the long-term consequences of SARS-CoV-2 on the brain. With technical guidance from the World Health Organization, this large team of interdisciplinary researchers will examine the underlying biology that may contribute to Alzheimer's and other dementias.

EVOLUTIONARY CUES

Underneath all of it, though, there's the ever-present hope that many principles might be distilled into one, that there might be a singular way to conceptualize the magnificent assault on our bodies. In many ways, Long Covid and these types of infection-associated chronic diseases haven't been solved because of how and where we are looking. The right observations haven't been performed to build the foundation of the scientific house yet.

"The problem is that the scientific method is not 'hypothesis, test' which is what the NIH does," Ron Davis says. "The actual scientific process is '*observation*, hypothesis, test.'" Charles Darwin didn't come up with the theory of evolution by sitting at his desk: "He went around and observed things, saw evolution actually happening, and then began to ask why. So that's why you don't want to sit and come up with a hypothesis in a very abstract way. You'd like it to be based on an observation, and sometimes the observation can be the nature of the disease, and ME/CFS affects so many different things. But you want to go deeper than that, and the best way to do that in my opinion is by collecting molecular data. Then ask why in the world is this high or low? Then you can begin to explore."

Starting something completely new is much harder than piggybacking off an existing research agenda—for instance, the data generated by ongoing cancer research offers fodder for future cancer grants. Incremental science is possible when there's a foundation from which to build. But the Human Genome Project had been different. It propelled a revolution in biology, stemming from a soaring strength that it didn't have a hypothesis. The giant data-gathering endeavor almost by definition had to be nothing more than an exercise in observation. There was no past agenda to build on. It was all brand new. With a map of every gene in the human body, scientists could later systematically discern what each of them might do.

Through the lens of genetics and molecular biology, diseases like Long Covid and ME/CFS take shape a bit differently as we tip into the substantial question of "why?" Genetics research begs to understand questions around evolution and selective pressure or why certain organisms have either a survival benefit or disadvantage. At first glance, this presents a paradox for disease states, especially ones where behavior is so greatly affected. Afterall, how could someone who is bedbound—unable to care for themselves let alone bear children—survive and successfully pass their genes onto the next generation? Perhaps the genetic mistake that allowed for an ME/CFS-like state to survive 100,000 years in humans doesn't manifest before childbearing age, therefore one might successfully pass their genes onto the next generation before succumbing to one's illness.

On the other hand, what advantage might chronic diseases give people in terms of survival?

Ron Davis suggests the disease state witnessed in conditions such as Long Covid or ME/CFS could have been caused by an organism needing to rest. He is convinced that there may be a set of genes that can trigger ME/CFS. From one point of view, there's an evolutionary basis that the sickness behavior triggered by an infectious agent is a signal for an organism to rest and allow the immune system to kick in and heal the organism. However, rather than serving as a temporary adaptive state, the system could shift for some reason into permanent dysfunction. Other animals, like bears, bees, and snakes, exhibit hibernation behavior and retreat into a power-down mode where only the essential bodily functions are maintained for long periods of time. This mode of operation allows the animal to survive extremely harsh conditions. University of California at San Diego researcher and Davis' collaborator Robert K. Naviaux found that people with ME/CFS show markedly slowed metabolism and suggests that this state is similar to a "dauer state" seen in nematode worms exposed to life-threatening conditions like starvation or toxins.

Although some animals bear resemblance to one another, Davis is suspicious of one transforming into a meaningful model of the disease. "I don't know if we'll ever find an animal model that is a decent model for ME/CFS. If a mouse comes down with ME/CFS it's only probably a matter of hours before it gets eaten," Davis said. In most cases, given an atmosphere in which only the fittest survive, natural selection would weed out those with disabilities who couldn't easily survive solely on their own. "We're a tribal sort of organism," he explained. "We'll take care of one other. That's been one of our strengths. We populated the world because of this intelligent way to take care of people, with a moral standard that we have to take care of everybody."

One thing is clear, despite our genes or because of them, humans are in a unique position to lean into our prosocial behavior as it surrounds the more vulnerable in our society. As Long Covid leaves millions with potentially lifelong physical and cognitive disabilities, it requires building out the social systems that take care of disabled people.

Chapter 14

A NEW EPIDEMIC OF DISABILITY

WITH MILLIONS OF PEOPLE EXPERIENCING long-term complications from Covid-19, the disease could cause decades of strain on our healthcare system, insurance industry, and federal safety net programs.

Figuring out exactly how Long Covid warps the economy and the labor market is a complex set of questions, which economists are only beginning to determine. The answer will be a function of how many people are sick, how sick they are, how long they stay sick, and the cost of medical interventions, assuming there are treatments that work. Finally, there's the cost of subsistence for families when Long Covid makes the primary wage earner too disabled to work. We do have some comparisons about the effect at scale. A 2015 study cited ME/CFS as causing an annual $17 to 24 billion impact on the U.S. economy in lost wages and inability to work.

In March 2021, the Body Politic's Fiona Lowenstein co-wrote a *New York Times* opinion piece with the PLRC's Hannah Davis. They argued that Long Covid could represent "one of the largest mass disabling events in modern history." The piece culminated what could be considered a trilogy of agenda-setting op-eds by Lowenstein, beginning with the piece telling the story of being hospitalized with Covid-19 at age twenty-six and the second article published a month later with the chronicle of prolonged recovery. This third essay, timed as the second year of the pandemic was getting underway, was prescient as well. Davis and Lowenstein benefitted from daily conversations with chronically ill patients whose lives were upended and could articulate a stark reality before it dawned on others. Public health authorities constantly reported on case counts, hospitalizations, and deaths. However, public dashboards displaying all kinds of pandemic data did not have any way of keeping track of how many people were failing to fully recover, the pair explained. The CDC didn't directly track that type of record.

For reference, polio was disabling about 35,000 people per year in the 1940s in the U.S. at a time when parents feared letting their children outside during the summer months. As of late April 2022, an estimated 81 million Americans had tested positive for the coronavirus, per the CDC's tracker. If a conservative 10 percent had symptoms lasting more than three months, that would mean nearly eight million had a chronic illness. If only 1 percent of them became disabled, that would indicate 800,000 Americans had been disabled within two years of the virus first being identified in China.

But the CDC knew from the PLRC's published study of Body Politic Slack group members that a large number of their members reported they hadn't been able to return to work, and many were being denied disability benefits.

British statistics offered a more detailed snapshot. Across the pond, British scientist Nisreen Alwan, an associate professor at the University of Southampton, had been campaigning with a similar pitch, expressed in the Twitter hashtag #CountLongCovid.

More than one in ten respondents reported symptoms twelve weeks after testing positive for Covid, according to a study by the nation's Office of National Statistics.

In its effort to track the post-acute sequelae of Covid, the American Academy of Physical Medicine and Rehabilitation eventually released its own PASC dashboard. On any given day, you could set the parameters on its dashboard for a given long-term symptom percentage rate. The algorithm then spits out how many new Covid long haulers were generated that day. If the total U.S. case count was 148,000, and the rate was 10 percent, then there were going to be 14,800 new Long Covid cases. But such a tool was a far cry from actionable information with its inputs based on estimates rather than a real-world count. Public health officials were largely blind because doctors and public health departments had no way of officially reporting Long Covid cases.

In June 2021, Davis and McCorkell presented the PLRC findings to a meeting of the White House Covid Health Equity Task Force. Among their recommendations was creating a federal short term disability program. A year of volunteer advocacy appeared to be paying off when the federal government recognized that Long Covid could be considered under the Americans with Disabilities Act.

"Many Americans who seemingly recover from the virus still face lingering challenges, like breathing problems, brain fog, chronic pain, and fatigue," President Joe Biden said in a Rose Garden speech, marking the thirty-first anniversary of the ADA.

"We're bringing agencies together to make sure Americans with Long Covid, who have a disability, have access to the rights and resources that are due under the disability law," he said.

In coordination, a host of executive branch agencies, including the Health and Human Services, the Department of Justice, and the Department of Labor, released their own guidance and resources supporting long haulers. This ensured that employers would be required to provide accommodations such as modified equipment or work schedules.

Biden touted the initiative as the "first of its kind" to address the new disease, designed for long haulers "so they can live their lives in dignity." The policies were largely a reiteration of existing law, but still the public acknowledgment from the White House was powerful, prompting a statement from Body Politic praising the move.

Lisa McCorkell, the public policy expert in the Patient-Led Research Collaborative, noted in the Body Politic statement that the official buy-in from the federal government would help reduce the "self-advocacy burden" long haulers felt in navigating access to accommodations and services.

Approval to receive full disability benefits through the Social Security Administration in the U.S. is a tall order. While some medical conditions offer instant approval, many aren't so easy. Proving that you qualify for disability means showing that your health condition has made, or is expected to make, it impossible to work for twelve months. Most applicants are denied on their first attempt. The U.S. doesn't offer a federal program for short-term disability benefits. Most European nations offer universal paid leave policies and more generous healthcare policies.

Absent a wonder drug, the most effective therapy for Long Covid and similar conditions is rest. Profound rest. That's not easy if you have to work in order to pay rent, care for elderly parents, or have young mouths to feed.

That's why McCorkell and the PLRC included a federal short-term disability plan in their presentation to the White House Covid Equity Task Force. Because exertion can worsen symptoms and lead to disability, essentially all the patients I spoke to for this book felt that those who had the relative privilege of resting for as long as possible—rather than being forced back to work—had at least a better shot of trying to prevent some of the worst harms the illness could inflict.

When physicians make a diagnosis they must plug in an insurance code, which all hail from the International Classification of Diseases (ICD). The system holds immense power because whether or not a doctor is willing to make a diagnosis can hinge on whether an insurance company will pay for a particular appointment or treatment. The specificity of the codes can get a bit absurd. For instance, there's the code W55.41XA, for "bitten by a pig, initial encounter." If you're struck by a duck, your doctor can file that under W61.62XD, and there are other codes if the offender is a cow or a macaw. If you happen to be injured in a spacecraft collision, that's V95.43XS. You're covered by a separate code if you get hit by a roller skater on the street. And it's hard to imagine what prompted the creation of a code for "burn due to water skis on fire, subsequent encounter," but your doctor's office can file a claim for you if it happens to you, too.

There were codes for suspected Covid exposure or for the rare multisystem inflammatory disease in children, but for more than a year, long haulers existed in a kind of bureaucratic no-man's land. On October 1, 2021, the ICD-10 code U09.9 went live, enabling reimbursement for "Post-Covid-19 condition, unspecified." The tweak vastly simplified the process by which patients navigated the labyrinthine insurance system and helped protect them from unexpected bills. Lisa McCorkell, from the Patient-Led Research Collaborative, ran point on representing Long Covid patients' interest in the discussions with the WHO and CDC.

Less than a week after the ICD-10 code rolled out, the World Health Organization published its case definition for "post-

Covid conditions," criteria which could be used universally for diagnostic or research purposes to identify who had the disease. This distinction matters, injecting authority and clarity into the pandemic fog of war. The WHO unified around a list of symptoms, including cognitive dysfunction, fatigue, and breathlessness, which lasted more than three months after the initial onset and had an impact on everyday functioning. Seventeen global experts had served on the WHO's working group, including the PLRC's Hannah Davis, filling the agency's new expert category of "patient-researcher."

Disease case definitions formalize whole scientific fields, ensuring everyone is referring to the same illness in the same way. When the definition was approved, some had lived with the symptoms fitting the criteria for fifteen months, a seeming eternity. But in the history of disease, the mobilization and consensus was lightning-fast. By contrast, a similar process for HIV/AIDS had required nearly four years, with the first human immunodeficiency virus case being identified in June 1981, researchers coalescing around the name of "acquired immune deficiency syndrome" in September 1982, and the WHO's AIDS case definition being released in October 1985.

AN UNREADY SAFETY NET

Patient advocates could shine a light on the new disease and help implement changes to healthcare systems, but the deterioration of their own bodies defied what bureaucracies were even capable of addressing.

For instance, after nineteen months without an income, Karyn Bishof, a co-founder of the Long Covid Alliance, was denied disability coverage for her Long Covid case at the end of September 2021.

The terse notice from the Social Security Administration stated, "While you are not capable of performing work you have done in the past, you are able to perform work that is less demanding." The single mom from Boca Raton, Florida disagreed. Given the variable nature of her unyielding symptoms, it was impossible to schedule a reliable hour or two in which she could work a job. Even if she could, she worried that attempting to work while so chronically ill would drive her health down below the basic motherly requirements of caring for her twelve-year-old son Jayani. There was no way of predicting when she would have physical ability or cogent thoughts. She hadn't been healthy enough to work for more than a year and a half after falling ill with Covid in the first wave. The timing of her illness was particularly cruel, coming after Bishof had completed two years of training to become a firefighter and paramedic. She had envisioned 2020 as a culmination of a lifelong dream that she'd put off for years as she raised her son. But it was not to be.

Prior to Covid, she worked out five days a week doing high-intensity interval training. Now she needed to spend as many as twenty hours a day in bed. She relied on her son to take their dog out, and to sweep, mop, wash dishes, and help with grocery shopping. Jayani was proud to contribute.

"Originally, before Covid, I did a fair amount, but I feel like I have a lot more responsibility now," he said. "I have to step up."

With Bishof's POTS symptoms, it was a titanic effort to walk upright for more than ten minutes before her heart rate skyrocketed and she had trouble staying conscious, so she and her son divided grocery store aisles between the two of them when they bought food. Some days she had to stay in the car while he made the rounds for her.

"I fight so hard so that I can also get better. But I'm really fighting for my son to have his mom because it really is just me and him in this whole world," she told me.

Bishof had thrived in the intense environment of firefighter training, pushing through injuries to graduate. But Long Covid was a vastly more brutal test of the body and soul. Among her dozens of symptoms were debilitating migraines that left her hiding under blankets for a day, insomnia that limited her sleep to a few hours each night, and inexplicable rashes on her arms. Constant nausea made it difficult to down her meds or eat more than one meal a day. When Bishof went out for doctor's appointments, she packed blankets and pillows in the car so she could rest before the drive home.

She couldn't earn her $55,000 salary. And she couldn't qualify for unemployment checks, because the program require certification that one is *capable* of working. She wasn't. With no one else to turn to, Bishof had to make do with food stamps as well as temporary cash assistance from the state of Florida that amounted to $158 per month. The cash assistance was still a few dollars short of paying the monthly power bill, and was thousands of dollars less than their other monthly expenses. Despite managing to raise a little over $2,000 online with a GoFundMe campaign, it wasn't enough, and being denied for disability meant falling one step further toward homelessness. In the coming months, there could be a lien on her house. It wasn't hard to envision the water or power being turned off, and she worried that child protective services might intervene to take her son.

"When I turn fourteen, I'm looking for jobs that I can do over the summer," Jayani, a seventh grader, told me. "I've been waiting to do a grocery store job where I'm a bag boy—I would be a really good bag boy—to just earn a little bit of income for us, because we don't get much income. No income at all really."

He played on a travel team where he'd met most of his closest friends, and he said he dreamed of becoming a professional soccer player. Given how high his civics grades were, and how much he liked reading history, his mom thought he ought to be a politician.

"You got to hope whoever's in charge of this actually wants to help," Jayani told me. "The long haulers aren't really being listened to. They all want this to be researched because it might be the key to getting rid of most of their stuff. I don't think there's going to be a cure for all of Long Covid, but I think there are going to be ways to bring it down so it's not as severe and there are ways to get people back to their normal lives."

If he did run for office one day, telling his mother's story of fighting through bureaucracy might carry the poetry of a stump speech that could win votes. There was heartbreaking irony in how Bishof, herself a national leader in the long hauler advocacy community, was falling through the cracks in the social safety net. That voluntary work, informed by her background studying health promotions and exercise science in college and fueled by a sense of desperation to get her own life back, carried the promise of benefiting millions of people.

Shortly after falling ill, Bishof created the Covid-19 Longhauler Advocacy Project. Later, she co-founded the Long Covid Alliance. Among her extensive list of contributions, she helped seed online support groups all over the country, built a comprehensive care guide for patients and medical providers, provided input to Congress for legislation to help long haulers, and consulted with the NIH as it designed its research initiatives for post-Covid conditions.

"I have a unique position in both being a patient, but also having health care experience and research experience. My background allows me to kind of take the best of both worlds—

the messaging of both worlds—and relay them to the other side," she said.

Knowing the long odds, Bishof had tried to be strategic, waiting to file her disability application until April 2021, once she could document a full twelve months of disability. She couldn't list all of her diagnoses in the online form, but she included her post-Covid conditions as postural orthostatic tachycardia syndrome, myalgic encephalomyelitis/chronic fatigue syndrome, fibromyalgia, chronic migraines, autoimmune disease, post-traumatic stress disorder, and Ehlers-Danlos syndrome. The notice from the SSA showed that the agency had received documentation from seven out of the more than twenty doctors Bishof had seen.

Because of the multisystem nature of her conditions, she needed care from a complex list of specialists—a rheumatologist, an endocrinologist, a migraine specialist, a geneticist, and a motility specialist, to name a few. Some had waiting lists as long as eight months. Her physicians collectively had made no progress in developing treatment plans. The delays in arriving at adequate care and the mounting medical bills left her under severe financial stress while she ate through her savings and her health worsened. She was caught up in a vicious cycle. She needed an attorney to be able to fight her case and win her appeal for disability with the Social Security Administration. But because she couldn't work, she couldn't afford to hire a lawyer. All of her energy for a whole day might be sucked up by a single phone call or one appointment. And even with an attorney, if her case required a hearing, that might mean waiting another year to get through the backlog of cases. Meanwhile her expertise within patient, medical, and policymaker communities didn't offer any tangible direction either.

"I don't know one person—one long hauler—who's been accepted for disability post-Covid," she said.

Unfortunately, it's not a surprise that Bishof and other long haulers like her would be denied the coverage. The program's eligibility criteria are notably stringent. The rolls are kept tight by design. The Social Security Disability Insurance program, created in 1956 under President Dwight Eisenhower, is funded by payroll taxes taken out of workers' paychecks each month. Applicants are required to have worked for at least a quarter of their adult lives and at least five of the last ten years. They must have medical documentation that they've already been disabled and incapable of gainful employment for at least twelve months or expect to be. And they must then endure a waiting period of another five months before receiving their determination. Decisions are based on medical documentation of an individual's functionality, regardless of diagnosis.

To be accepted, applicants must show that they can't perform "substantial gainful activity," meaning they are unable to hold down a job earning $1,350 monthly, or $16,200 annually. And still, those who do qualify aren't winning a golden ticket: Nine in ten beneficiaries receive $2,000 or less per month, consigning them to a life below the federal poverty level and short of affording market rate rent. Those criteria—which put the U.S. among the strictest of developed nations—mean that just 34 percent of applicants ultimately win benefits, either on their first try or on their appeal, according to the Center on Budget and Policy Priorities.

Further, poverty rates and ill health are still high among those denied coverage, according to a 2014 analysis published in the *Journal of Disability Policy Studies*, a fact that reinforces how strict the requirements truly are. Most people who do end up qualifying for benefits are so significantly disabled that they'll stay on the program for life. So far, Bishof felt like she was just a statistic in a larger tidal wave of disability threatening to overload the system.

"I wish that I could say that it would happen sooner rather than later. But I think it's gonna come years down the road when they start realizing how so many people unable to work affects the economy," she told me. "And I think that they're going to unfortunately only care about Long Covid when it comes down to the numbers versus the experiences of those people."

If a substantial number of Covid long haulers don't recover and return to work, the sheer size of their population represents a substantial risk to the workforce. In 2020, just over 8 million U.S. workers were Social Security disability beneficiaries. With the median age of Long Covid occurring around middle age, the heart of the disease burden falls on people at the prime of their working lives.

LONG HAULERS DISRUPT THE SYSTEM

"Covid long haulers represent the largest influx of new entrants to the disability community in modern history," according to Rebecca Vallas, a senior fellow at the Century Foundation. "Evidence suggests that between three million and ten million Americans may now have Long Covid. These are just wildly, wildly large numbers for a system that is already not handling the existing population seeking to access these benefits. This is a system that wasn't prepared even before the pandemic."

Vallas began her career in the 2000s as a legal aid attorney in Philadelphia representing people who had been denied disability benefits right out of law school. The job left a mark on her. She had to counsel her low-income clients that being denied on the first attempt was part of the system. "The human consequences are absolutely dire," she explained. Without an income, disabled people often exhausted their savings, lost their homes when they couldn't pay mortgages, and could be reduced to living out of their cars.

"Thousands of people die every single year when they are waiting for disability benefits," she said. "Those are statistics that might be a gut punch at one level when you hear them in the abstract, but I saw this firsthand more times than I can count—and certainly more times than I would like to remember—during my legal aid days because I was representing someone who didn't have enough resources to meet human survival needs."

Those experiences motivated her to become an advocate working on public policy reform in Washington. Working for the Center for American Progress, she helped launch the think tank's Disability Justice Initiative, and frequently testified in front of Congress about disability and poverty issues, working to defend the SSA from budget cuts.

"I can tell you we have made it incredibly, incredibly difficult to access what are literally survival benefits," she told me. "We make people jump through a maze of Kafkaesque hoops and fill out a mountain of paperwork that honestly is complex even for lawyers. And all of that is to access incredibly modest benefits."

Add to that the fact that during the pandemic, the SSA's 1,200 field offices were closed—blocking access for on-demand or walk-in services of particular need for those with low incomes, no incomes, mental health issues, or limited English proficiency needing to file applications and fix bureaucratic errors. It contributed to historically unprecedented declines of 25 percent fewer people receiving benefits across all disabilities.

For Covid long haulers, though, the process could seem even more impossible. Some people did present with specific, concrete, anatomical damage that could be verified with objective medical documentation. But there wasn't a basic blood test for Long Covid that could furnish that type of objective proof to SSA's satisfaction. Even if patients could find a specialist who understood the condition, they were often jam-packed and overbooked.

"One of the opportunities of this moment is a paradigm shift when it comes to how our society understands the concept of disability. That's true in the disability system as we're talking about how many are wrongfully denied because they don't fit into the Social Security Administration's mold for how they recognize disability," Vallas told me. "But that's true even more broadly, given that we have for so long portrayed disability as a person in a wheelchair or with a physical disability. Now we've got chronic illness in the spotlight in a way that has not happened in quite some time, if ever, at this scale. And we have a paradigm shift away from disbelief and gaslighting. We should move away from a program that's designed to deny people and been so defined by the 'makers, takers, fakers' mythology towards one that is intended to be there for people in their time of need, and, dare I say, that is actually accessible."

One way Vallas and disability advocates hoped to improve access was through setting up a "navigators" program to help people find their way through the byzantine system, similar to those created by the Affordable Care Act for buying health insurance in the marketplace. Another area of low hanging fruit for reform would be to pass legislation eliminating the mandatory five-month waiting period to receive SSDI benefits and the additional twenty-four-month period recipients must wait before they can obtain health coverage through Medicare. And even adjusting programs for inflation—and tagged to the federal poverty level—would be a step up from the status quo. If people could get approved from day one, without needing to wait years to win an appeal at a hearing, then they could dodge at least some of the descent into poverty and have a better shot at a dignified life.

As many as 1.6 million jobs in the U.S. could be unfilled due to Long Covid, according to an analysis by Katie Bach, a non-resident senior fellow at the Brookings Institution. After a year and a half of pandemic, hordes of workers quit their jobs, in a steady mass migration seeking out new opportunities that would become known as the Great Resignation. The result was a historic U.S. labor shortage, an unusual economy characterized not by too few jobs, but by too few workers. Many were pursuing better working conditions or seeking out new dreams.

But 31 million working-age Americans were likely somewhere on the spectrum of Long Covid, either with some lingering symptoms or a more intense disabling illness. Therefore, about 15 percent of the ongoing workforce problem could be due to long haulers unable to continue working or who needed to work fewer hours due to their illness or disability, she argued, citing the PLRC's peer-reviewed research showing that about a quarter of long haulers in their study were no longer working. To be conservative, Bach assumed that a third of Long Covid patients stayed sick for about three months, such that as many as 4.5 million long haulers were sick at any given time during the pandemic. If about a quarter of them couldn't work, that meant that at any point some 1.1 million Americans were not working due to Long Covid. Further, another study had showed that 46 percent long haulers had needed to reduce their hours at work, enlarging the impact to 1.6 million full-time equivalent workers.

Getting an accurate snapshot of the actual labor impact is a question encumbered by the instruments that economists use to collect data. Just as there are limits in how quickly biomedical science can ask the right questions and publish quality literature about a new disease, economists also have their hands tied in trying to immediately characterize the sheer mass pall that condition casts across individual lives and fortunes. Building those questions into surveys is the most robust way to ensure long haulers get counted from a labor perspective. The most responsive tool is the U.S. Census Bureau's Household Pulse Survey, a twenty-minute online questionnaire, Bach explains. Its question structure asking about employment status doesn't carve out a space to specifically capture Long Covid as the reason for not working, giving respondents an option to say they were sick with coronavirus symptoms, or that they are sick or disabled with something other than the coronavirus. The average Long Covid patient would likely feel that either of those categories didn't apply to them. The Census Bureau's monthly Current Population Survey, a more rigorous assessment, has a similar issue in that long haulers might fall through the cracks.

Bach advocated for the Census Bureau to work with the NIH research teams and patient advocacy groups to write questions that could meaningfully collect information on the number of people disabled by Long Covid, the average time not working or needing reduced hours, the workplace accommodations they would need to get back to work.

"Until we have data from a representative sample that accurately capture the extent of the impacts to the labor force, economists and policymakers are likely not going to consider Long Covid an economic issue or recognize it for the mass disabling event that it is," Lisa McCorkell said.

In April 2022, a team of researchers organized by the Solve Long Covid Alliance published a white paper with the most thorough estimate yet of Long Covid's economic impact to the U.S. It based its assumptions off data that between 7 million and

14 million Americans, amounting to 2.3 percent and 4.4 percent of the population respectively, had experienced or were experiencing disabling Long Covid through January 2022. If so, the total impact to the U.S. economy ranged from $386 billion to $511 billion, as the disease prevented many from returning to the workforce as their previous selves.

The researchers argued that the mass disabling event highlighted the a "need for changes to the structure of U.S. disability benefit programs as demand exponentially increases." Postviral disability was not an immutable state. The disability caused by Long Covid was waxing and waning, such that employees might be capable of working one day and incapable the next. They called for disability benefits systems to recognize partial disability. Further, they called for systems to drop caps on earnings, which counterproductively can create barriers preventing those who are capable of working from entering back into the workforce part-time or with accommodations during periods in which their symptoms were less severe. Creating a stable post-Covid workforce meant providing incentives for employers and employees to work together to support rehabilitation of workers with post-Covid health conditions and to accommodate the large number of workers likely to be experiencing disabilities.

That number of workers affected was jaw-dropping, in part because it was in range with the total number of workers, 8 million, who had lost their jobs during the lowest parts of the Great Recession in 2008. If the totally amount of disability veered toward the higher end of their projection, then the resulting socioeconomic impact would be "seismic" in scope.

Chapter 15

THE ePATIENT REVOLUTION AND CROWDSOURCING RESEARCH

SUSANNAH FOX WAS ONE OF the people most stunned by the resilience and resourcefulness of Long Covid patients.

"We are watching patients, caregivers, clinicians, researchers, and policymakers move through the stages of peer-to-peer health innovation at a fast clip," she wrote in a blog post about Long Covid patient activism in January 2021. "Faster than I've ever seen in my twenty years of tracking this phenomenon."

She is the type of person you'd want to impress, as someone who is uniquely qualified to spot patients changing the world. From 2015 to 2017, Fox had led health innovation efforts as the Chief Technology Officer for the U.S. Department of Health and Human Services. She rose to that position after a career charting the ways people diagnosed with life-altering diseases had built and leveraged online communities to share hard-won wisdom not available anywhere else, track symptoms, pool their data, and generally take back control of their own destinies.

She was used to seeing a specific storyline across diseases. Patients began with feeling isolated and alone. Then they discover a group, develop a sense of identity or pride with their new community, and then eventually spearhead a project to fix what they perceive as broken in a health system. Here, she was seeing a group innovating before the world even knew the condition existed.

During her time in the federal government, Fox had been impressed by the work of the Cajun Navy, an informal group of volunteers and boat owners who banded together to rescue people stranded in their homes following devastating flooding in the aftermath of Hurricanes Katrina and Harvey. Credited with saving thousands of lives, they served in areas where the government's emergency response was spread too thin. Their heroism prompted the Federal Emergency Management Agency to coordinate with them as part of a whole community approach to disaster response.

As Covid-19 tore through society and misinformation became rampant, Fox wondered if a digital health version of the Cajun Navy could activate in support of pandemic response, particularly with a citizen brigade who could help aid not just in disseminating accurate scientific information about the virus, but also in building tools to help patients track symptoms, pointing people in the right direction to get care, and even organizing the science themselves. Just as the Cajun Navy blurred the line between citizen and first responder, she thought there could be a similar model for tapping into people's existing skill sets to enlist them directly in public health. In particular, those who had been infected themselves might have the most useful firsthand experience to offer others newly getting sick. The answer was in organic peer-to-peer health communities, and the PLRC was the most effective version she had ever seen.

Fox's life story made her perfectly poised to understand the significance of what they had accomplished. A self-described "Internet geologist," Fox was instrumental in creating the original website for *US News and World Report* in 1995, eventually working her way up to becoming its lead online editor. She then spent a decade and a half with the Pew Research Center, helping start its Internet and American Life Project focusing on health and technology.

Early in that role, around the turn of the millennium, she met Dr. Tom Ferguson, a Yale-trained physician who believed in the power of patients to contribute not just to their own well-being, but to scientific discovery as well. Though he had never practiced medicine, he wrote prolifically, serving as the medical editor of the counterculture magazine *Whole Earth Catalog* and representing a strain of self-sufficiency within the hippie movement. Its articles focused on how to build your own house, plant your own garden, and nurture your own health to prevent disease. Once you were diagnosed with a serious disease, self-reliance became less possible because doctors had a huge information advantage in the days before the Internet. Ferguson championed a more equal doctor-patient relationship. He felt doctors ought to collaborate with patients, rather than command them. He coined the term "e-patient" to describe empowered or expert patients who didn't just take greater control of their own healthcare but who actively built new platforms or communities or devices that could change the larger system.

HANGING OUT WITH COWBOYS AND REBELS TO SEE THE FUTURE FASTER

Ferguson's concepts would come to fuel the rest of Fox's career. Her research leveraged the power of Pew's research methodology to get a broad view of the national population. That data outlined details such as the number of households with Internet access or which types of people searched for health information online. She combined that with field work in which she interviewed members of early online patient communities.

"I would go into a certain patient community and spend time interviewing people, in order to stay in touch with what was being created, what was being built by these pioneers, by these rebels," she told me. "They were often left out of the main-stream conversation about health care because they were living with something rare or life-changing."

She got to know a host of digital health pioneers, including the founder of Psych Central, the first mental health website.

"I began generating reports focused on the evolution of the digital health culture and market every two years. And Tom [Ferguson] was my guide," she told me. "What Tom taught me is that if you hang out with the cowboys and rebels and pioneers, you will see the future faster."

Many of those people weren't typical tech geeks. They plunged into online communities out of sheer desperation. Some of the most avid early adopters of technology were those who were trying to save their own lives or the lives of their children.

"I would learn from these radical patient communities, and I would bring that back and ask questions to start tracking the trends," she said. "It's through them that I saw the real future of healthcare, which is bringing it back into the home, allowing people who are kitchen table innovators to contribute to science and to contribute to medical and assistive device innovation."

As the Internet matured, patients and caregivers developed increasingly sophisticated ways to use digital technology as a tool to share real-world knowledge about treatments and accelerate research or even self-organize their own studies. One key step in the unfolding of the ePatient movement was the launch of the site PatientsLikeMe, founded in 2005. Brothers Jamie and Ben Heywood started the platform in honor of their brother Stephen who was diagnosed with amyotrophic lateral sclerosis in 1998, at the age of twenty-nine. The neurodegenerative disease, commonly known as ALS, famously afflicted baseball great Lou Gehrig and astrophysicist Stephen Hawking, and it can begin with a muscle twitching or weakness in the limbs. It leads to full-body paralysis, affecting the muscles needed to eat, speak, breathe, and eat. It has no known cure and results in death.

Desperate to save or at least prolong Stephen's life, the brothers became citizen scientists, consuming every bit of research and literature they could find about ALS. One of the best resources that could serve their purpose, though, didn't really exist yet. They wanted to mine insights from a trove of data about the lived experiences of others with the disease. For the brothers, that meant building a set of tools on the PatientsLikeMe site—as well as a community of patients using them—to crowdsource that information themselves.

"What PatientsLikeMe offered was an opportunity to at least track data so that the ALS patients together could start to understand the trajectory of the disease in ways that no clinical registry gave them access to," Fox said.

In one example, a small trial in Italy in 2008 showed that the drug lithium carbonate might have an effect on slowing the progression of ALS. That glimmer of hope prompted patients from all over the world to use PatientsLikeMe to self-organize a larger observational study using self-reported data from 348 users on the site. After twelve months the trial ultimately did not show that lithium carbonate was effective in combating the disease, but the way in which the patients had rallied toward finding an answer became a parable for how exasperated patients, who did not have time to wait for traditional scientific methodology, could take research into their own hands. If you're going to be dead before scientists can deliberate about a new standard of care, you've got to invent a new process.

Today, PatientsLikeMe boasts a community of more than 850,000 users representing nearly 3,000 different health conditions, and a track record of generating more than 100 peer-reviewed papers for patients with various diseases.

Another one of the "cowboys" in patient-led innovation was Dave deBronkart, a fifty-six-year-old Boston man working in tech marketing, who was diagnosed with stage IV kidney cancer in 2007. The condition carried a median survival time of just twenty-four weeks. His doctor "prescribed" him an online patient community, the Association of Cancer Online Resources, at ACOR.org, a story deBronkart tells in his 2011 TEDx talk. When he joined the group, he met patients who told him about an uncommon treatment, high-dosage interleukin, not offered in most hospitals and for which there wasn't any information available through government websites. The therapy had only a slim chance of helping, but for deBronkart, that was still vastly preferable to the alternative. He didn't want to ask his daughter and her boyfriend to get "married prematurely, just so you can do it while dad's still alive," he explained to the crowd. The patient experts on ACOR sent him the phone numbers for a few physicians in his area who could prescribe the treatment. It worked: the tumor sizes shrank dramatically when he received the treatments, each two months apart. DeBronkart witnessed his daughter's wedding a year and a half later. He is alive today in 2022 because of a patient community.

But his story accelerated from there. DeBronkart believed that his own experience could serve as part of a greater hive mind and be used to benefit others. If he and other patients could aggregate their anonymized data together, then smart software could comb through it to find patterns that could help lead to early detection or treatments for diseases, including the cancer that had nearly killed him. DeBronkart authorized his hospital to transfer his data to Google Health, which was experimenting with a project by which users could volunteer their health records from various sources to create a central health profile with all their conditions, medications, and lab results in one place. But when he downloaded his electronic health record from the hospital that had saved his life, he found it rife with errors, because the hospital transferred the billing codes rather than his clinical data. That brought up a more fundamental question of whether patients could fully entrust their health to any institution. If medical record data came from patients' own bodies and was collected to further their own health, should they be allowed to have sovereignty over it? DeBronkart's story ended up on the front page of the *Boston Globe* in April 2009.

The ensuing attention catapulted him into a prolific new career as a cancer blogger, speaker, and patient rights activist. That summer, when the organizer of the Medicine 2.0 conference called to ask him the theme of his keynote later that year, deBronkart said, "Gimme my damn data, because you can't be trusted." That phrase became a rallying call for greater patient engagement in transforming the health system. He was elected co-chair of the Society for Participatory Medicine. Known affectionately as "e-Patient Dave," he became one of the most recognized figures in the e-patient movement, evangelizing a mantra that patients are the most underused resource in healthcare.

A few years later, in 2012, another crowdsourced medical platform, called CrowdMed, was formed. As the name suggests, CrowdMed crowd sources knowledge from both health professionals and self-proclaimed citizen "medical detectives" to diagnose challenging and rare disease cases. After debuting its beta testing in Washington, D.C. at TEDMED in 2013, CrowdMed has gone on to raise $2.4 million from investors and worked on more than 1,000 cases. A patient can choose one of three packages and upload their own story, including how the disease has affected their life holistically. Medical detectives might be medical students, curious doctors, patients, or other interested parties. The top three diagnoses are chosen and the detectives can be up-ranked by patient feedback and previous correct diagnoses. The company points to its relatively cheap access to medical knowledge and its self-serve, patient-centered interface as innovations. While some worry about the reliability of the suggested diagnoses being provided, satisfied patients and founder Jared Heyman maintain that when looking for a diagnosis to a challenging or rare disease, many heads are better than one.

Fox explains that getting society to accept a new idea means first fighting back against a prevailing belief that the idea is radically crazy, borrowing a concept from *Wired* magazine co-founder Kevin Kelly's essay "The Natural History of a New Idea." First, the idea is outright wacko, then it's simply odd but unproven. If it has staying power, people begin to see it as true, but insignificant. Finally, in the fourth stage, an idea is simply *obvious*, something all of us knew all along. The framework can be applied to virtually an infinite number of phenomena, from the laws of gravity and the existence of the Americas, onward to the abolition of slavery and the rise of the most recent presidential candidate. The notion that Covid-19 could cause long-term illness might follow a similar rise into the public and scientific consciousness. In this case, Fox said, the progression would be "Crazy. Crazy. Long Covid. Obvious."

She took note of how Body Politic and the Patient-Led Research Collaborative were helping the whole health ecosystem respond quickly to what seemed to many to be a new post-viral syndrome. She reached out to get in touch and help however she could.

"They're super conscious that they're standing on the shoulders of giants, that so many people built things that they are benefiting from," Fox said.

They were a perfect embodiment of how she conceived a peer health innovation pipeline, beginning with a person afflicted with new symptoms and feeling isolated and alone. Finding an online patient community led to connection with others experiencing the same roadblocks and then brainstorming with them about what to do in spite of those issues. Pretty soon the groups were tapping into their existing skills as entrepreneurs to build a solution. Companies, researchers, and government agencies could then partner with the self-organized communities to amplify their signal or scale up a product or process that seemed to support sufferers or treat the disease.

DESIGNING A PATIENT-CENTERED FUTURE

I had first become aware of Fox after I produced *Forgotten Plague* and was selected as an "ePatient Scholar" to attend the Stanford Medicine X conference in 2014. I had no idea of the tradition into which I was entering. On stage, she told stories of how she had led health innovation efforts at the top level of the federal government. I was a barely employed twenty-four-year-old, not long out of college, trying to tell the story of a disease most people had never heard of. Like many, I was managing a flare up of my illness that made it hard to sit through many of the sessions. I spent hours laying in the conference's "wellness" room, which was specifically designed with the knowledge that many of the patients needed that space in order to attend at all.

But I was thrilled to find my tribe of other idealists from across the spectrum of disease attempting their own piece in what the community touted as the "patient-centered revolution" in healthcare. There was Emily Kramer-Golinkoff, in her thirties with late-stage cystic fibrosis, who has now raised $10 million to support potentially life-saving research into her rare form of the disease and been named a White House Champion of Change. Another ePatient, Hugo Campos, also received that honor for his effort to claim ownership of the data in the device embedded in his heart for hypertrophic cardiomyopathy, which delivers a life-saving electric shock if (and when) the disease sends him into cardiac arrest. I also met Julie Flygare, who developed narcolepsy in law school before going on to write a memoir about the condition and build a non-profit organization that awards scholarships to students with narcolepsy. Their stories, too numerous to list, filled my cup, spurring me into a bolder vision.

Our group of several dozen ePatient Scholars was given reserved seating in the front rows and the majority of the priority speaking slots, which were staged with all the majesty and vulnerability of a TED event. Each ePatient was doing seemingly impossible work to rebuild or reform medicine in ways that centered and celebrated the human experience of illness.

Susannah Fox had been one of the earliest voices driving the creation of the Medicine X conference and the dynamic community it would come to foster. I came to believe the values invigorating its collective spirit carry tremendous power in forging the future of medicine.

At the core of Medicine X was a vision of Everyone Included™. This trademarked leadership and design framework embodies the notion that implementing change requires co-creation with patients, caregivers, providers, technologists, and researchers. So much of medicine can falter when it is siloed across huge institutions, and when stakeholders can't join the same conversation to brainstorm, build, and execute together. A tech company could build the most beautiful symptom-tracking app but it wouldn't matter if patients found it burdensome to input data or if it collected data that researchers couldn't use. Everyone Included is a moral acknowledgment of inherent human rights. Patients deserve a co-equal role in designing every aspect of the healthcare experience.

Distilled into ten design principles, Everyone Included means:

> *Be a rebel.*
> *Value each person.*
> *Be human.*
> *Be human-centered.*
> *Co-design.*
> *Facilitate connections.*
> *Treat with dignity.*
> *Provide a stage.*
> *Be beautiful and tasteful.*
> *Create magic.*

The Med X community radiated with "design thinking," a methodology for creative problem solving that celebrated radical collaboration. It has deep roots in Silicon Valley, particularly through the IDEO design firm, which built the first computer mouse for Apple. Design thinking prizes human-centered thinking, collective idea generation, rapid prototyping, and continuous testing of ideas to refine solutions to complex problems. Design thinking suffused the university through Stanford's "d School" (officially the Hasso Plattner Institute of Design), which exists to teach creative design principles to graduate students from across all of the university's disciplines, unlocking creative potential in everyone, whether they be journalists or engineers or educators or doctors.

The process begins by empathizing with the problem through stories to get to the emotional heart of the problem and define what needs to be solved. For instance, I participated in one design workshop over three days where the question was, "How might we improve access to pulmonary rehab for those with chronic obstructive pulmonary disease?" My view of the problem pivoted after being moved by long conversations with COPD patients participating in the program who explained how the disease altered the fabric of their daily lives. Then in the ideation phase, we, as designers, suspended judgment while brainstorming bold ideas regardless of their cost, absurdity, or even simplicity. Each little group in the workshop used black markers to write out ideas on yellow sticky notes as fast as possible. Next, the prototyping phase involves role playing or drawing up a storyboard with stick figures in a cartoon scene. In the COPD example, we explored how pulmonary rehab is the gold standard for treating the disease. But at a time in which rural hospitals are closing, centers offering the expensive service aren't reimbursed enough to be able to stay open. One solution we came up with was to create a national certification program whereby LA Fitness or Gold's Gym might offer the service. Another idea the dozens of us in the workshop fleshed out was to explore setting up pulmonary rehab in Walmart stores, similar to how the retailer offers optometry at its locations. From there, you test out the prototype, take extensive feedback, and assess how to iterate.

This was the tradition that the Patient-Led Research Collaborative was stepping into when they collectively produced the first research into the long-term effects of Covid-19. Their contribution could set the standard as a model for patient innovators to follow for other diseases as well. In June 2021, the group received a quarter-million dollar grant from the Patient-Centered Outcomes Research Institute, a federal agency created as part of the 2010 Affordable Care Act. PCORI was tasked with helping ensure patients and the public have information they can use to make healthcare decisions. In conjunction with the Council of Medical Specialty Societies, the PLRC was to explore how to bring their approach to other diseases, showcasing how to integrate patient-led research into clinical registries and formal research, building an ecosystem directly around the questions and treatment outcomes that mattered most to patients.

In their grant, they argued their model would light the way for a new paradigm in how patients could "move from research contributors to leaders of survey and research design."

And in April 2022, the PLRC received another shot in the arm in their mission to flip the script and forge a new future patient-centered care. They won a $3 million grant from Balvi, a fund created by Vitalk Buterin, the founder of the cryptocurrency Ethereum. Balvi sought high-impact Covid projects that could enable key research to be fast-tracked, and to end the pandemic. The new funding allowed the PLRC to fund full-time positions for its team of multi-disciplinary volunteer researchers who up to that point had needed to work unpaid or outside of their normal jobs for two years in order to press the international cases that Long Covid presented a severe public health problem. And it enabled the group to set up a Long Covid biomedical research fund led by patients, designed to accelerate knowledge of the underlying causes and treatments for Long Covid. They aimed to run a study on Covid reinfections, a quality of life study in a middle-income country, a phenotyping project, and a quarterly publication of patient-generated hypotheses shared in the public domain for Long Covid researchers to pursue.

Their mission to prove that patients were the experts in their own care was starting to look like it had staying power.

Chapter 16

EXPECTANT HOPE

DURING THIS SECOND COVID WINTER, I've retreated again to my parents' house to write. A year ago, I was sick in their basement fending off phone calls from disability insurance representatives, cycling through treatments, and desperately trying to carve out time to "recover." But even when I went back to work two months later, many of the residual symptoms remained. Within a few weeks, I was assigned to write a story exploring the early social media reports last spring that long haulers were improving after receiving the vaccine. As I began my research, I scheduled my first vaccine appointment immediately, hoping the shot might cure me as well. Riding up an escalator to the vaccination center within Atlanta's Mercedes-Benz Stadium, the atmospherics of an NFL game felt like a triumphal end to sickness. Yet the shots didn't wipe away the remaining symptoms—I still felt the strange buzzing sensations, the lack of energy, the loss of my usual ability to focus. I was well enough to travel to Colombia and Mexico with friends in the saddle period between waves when it seemed the virus' grip on our lives might be receding. However, other parts of me have yet to return. Each time I try going for a run or long bike ride, I feel sick for days afterwards.

The classic post-exertional malaise thwarts my ability to exercise and quiet my anxiety in a world gone mad.

But as long as I don't push it, my dad and I can go on long walks to discuss scientists I'm interviewing and to hash out the next round of edits. My mom watches medical lectures with me about the latest research discoveries, and we play a nightly game of ping pong. Writing this book has fulfilled few of my writerly fantasies of living like Henry David Thoreau in a cabin at Walden Pond, communing with a world spirit. I feel trapped. I'm mortally afraid of reinfection, knowing viscerally the pain that awaits if I go out for dinner with the wrong person or attend a party at times when it can sometimes seem that every other person is a carrier. With my body's low natural killer cell function, I worry that the next hit, if it happens, might be as bad, or worse, than the last. At least for now, taking shelter in this expansive house has been a refuge away from the dystopian timeline unfolding just outside.

Omicron and its lineage and sublineage variants have triggered massive new waves of Covid all over the world, and they will not be the last. We'll likely live with more waves for many years into the future. Though this most recent strain is perceived as "mild," its transmissibility is far beyond its predecessors. Its relative mildness is little consolation when hospitalizations are again overwhelming an already burned-out healthcare system and Long Covid most frequently stems from those with mild cases that never needed hospitalization in the first place. The first U.S. Omicron cases were identified during the first week of December 2021. By March 2022, there's little formal data to show how many people are getting sick with Omicron and developing long-term symptoms. But in late December 2021, Dr. Anthony Fauci reiterated that the proportion of those infected to those who develop Long Covid, 10 to 30 percent, is likely to remain steady. And every expert I've spoken with tells me that the new variant is only going to lead to another large wave of long haulers. Several leaders of online Long Covid support groups told me by early 2022 they were already seeing surges of new members into their communities. At least now some of the pioneering work has already been done. The virus has punctured modernity, and the continuous game of cat and mouse between variants and vaccines remains a birthing ground for long haulers.

Nearly every week, substantive new research findings are released, building an ever-stronger set of insights into the pathophysiological basis for Long Covid. We now have good evidence that Long Covid is more likely in individuals who create low levels of antibodies after the infection or who have autoantibodies, Epstein-Barr virus activation, or a history of type 2 diabetes.

In the U.S., Amy Proal, Akiko Iwasaki, and David Putrino have partnered in a global effort with Resia Pretorius of South Africa, Dr. Asad Khan in the UK, and Dr. Beate Jaeger of Germany to chase down the microclot story. This gives a convincing picture of at least one key facet of Long Covid.

"We're seeing a biomarker, the microclots, that is present in all of the patients we've tested so far," Putrino said. "Everyone has microclots that we've tested in varying degrees, and we're seeing measures of microclot load correlate with Long Covid clinical symptoms that I'm measuring, which is the first time that I've seen that very cleanly. I can correlate your cognitive scores with your clot scores."

So far, those studies have been small and needed to be repeated in much larger proportions. And removing the clots through an apheresis technique doesn't eliminate the underlying cause. Patients tested for the clots again after forty-eight hours show evidence of the clots reforming. Although the clots correlate with symptoms and may be causing the symptoms, some other upstream source is contributing to the clots. But still, the strength of the ongoing research gives him confidence that the apheresis technique could advance toward a randomized control trial and eventually multi-site studies.

"In the meantime, everything we're doing on the apheresis side is very much patient-led and patient-sanctioned, so we have people with Long Covid every step of the way telling us the way to do things that is appropriate for their population and their community," Putrino said. "My mantra hasn't changed since pre-Covid which is 'fail fast' on all these interventions. I want a quick yes or a quick no. Should we move on to the next phase or un-sentimentally start all over again?"

In other preprint studies, they found that specific cytokines correlated with particular symptoms, for instance the chemo-kine CCL11 being strongly associated with patients who complained of brain fog. But many of the markers so far are person-specific or symptom-specific, so they require a personalized medicine approach. And large quantities of virus were found in the GI tracts of individuals with GI symptoms in the acute phase of Covid, showing that SARS-CoV-2 was in fact capable of infecting the GI tract. For those with Long Covid whose illness is directly driven by persistent viral infection, those sorts of findings could offer the cleanest explanation. Trials to test out Pfizer's coronavirus antiviral Paxlovid in Long Covid could be a promising area of research to knock out viral reservoirs.

There will likely be better answers, perhaps even before this book is released. In the meantime, learning to forge a new life in spite of the hardship—inside of its limits—becomes not just its own kind of medical intervention, but actually a philosophical one as well.

HONING RESILIENCE

Apart from receiving an actual successful biomedical treatment, one of the most important principles for managing or healing from a new chronic illness is radical acceptance. Many people have a hard time getting better because they don't fully acknowledge how sick they really are. It can require a full stop in life, and a total reappraisal of the magnitude of the shift in our abilities. Allowing for a period of profound rest, as contrary as that may be to our modern obsession with productivity, is likely going to pay dividends years later if you can stop the disease's progress early in its tracks. Further, you must pursue an aggressive, and holistic, set of treatments that take into account how Long Covid, or any post-viral illness, has affected many different systems of your body rather than just one.

Forgive yourself if you're not able to do work or go to activities that used to be part of your life. Let yourself rest if you need it.

In a world where the science is changing or even the mere existence of one's disease is contested, self-advocacy becomes the one true north star. There are principles that you can follow to understand how to direct your own care or be the empowered expert in your own disease. Doctors don't have time to process every new study on Long Covid, and they obviously will not have learned about the disease in medical school. But by being a responsible student of the scientific literature, you can engage with your medical care in ways that doctors appreciate. Rather than conceiving of the doctor-patient relationship as paternalistic, you can strive to work with your doctor as a co-equal partner in your care.

Karyn Bishof assembled a list of resources on the Covid-19 Longhauler Advocacy Project site to help long haulers and their medical providers "work as a team in an attempt to get the patient back to good health and regain quality of life." Know that getting the outcomes you or a loved one need means partnering not just with physicians, but with whole healthcare ecosystems of nurses, social workers, and insurance representatives. Simply committing to staying organized with all the medical paperwork and insurance claims can make a huge difference in getting results smoothly to improve your health.

To best help busy health providers do their jobs, Bishof recommends building a binder to "pre-load" your doctor with information ahead of time. This can tell your story chronologically so that the whole appointment isn't spent reviewing lab work. Include a list of all your symptoms in order by severity of which affect your daily life most significantly. Compile a spreadsheet stating all your symptoms and activities over a two-week period, and paint a vivid picture of your quality of life or level of disability. Have a list of which additional tests you'd like ordered and which treatments you'd like to try. Get a friend to help you compile the info.

Make sure you take detailed notes during your appointment. If you're too sick, have a healthier friend, relative, or patient advocate accompany you to the appointment to listen and advocate for you. If you're not getting the care you need, fire your doctor and find a better one.

Long hauler Sandhya Kamphampati advised keeping track of all your data in a spreadsheet, which was her natural inclination as a data journalist. That way "I always had a log of everything I needed to track, especially my heart rate and oxygen, which, as a Long Covid patient, are helpful markers to share with my doctor," she wrote in the *Los Angeles Times*.

When the disease is loosely defined or research is scarce, you ought to bring supporting information such as studies, news articles, info posters or other resources to appointments. When the CDC released its interim post-Covid treatment guidelines in June 2021, it was essentially creating resources that patients could print out and show their doctors in order to direct them toward the recommended tests, procedures, or specialty clinics. For post-Covid patients who don't have a positive PCR test, the most useful part is the official word that Long Covid clinics shouldn't use any particular lab test as a make-or-break admission ticket to a clinic, providing coverage for a vast swath who might not otherwise have been able to get care.

One early stop can be the Job Accommodation Network, which offers free and confidential guidance on issues related to disability and employment. Accommodations can vary widely depending on the job. For instance, with remote work cultures becoming more accepted during the pandemic, it may be much easier to request arrangements to work from home or to lie down while working. There are basic adjustments that can ease some of the stress of working with a disability, such as using an ergonomic keyboard or dictation software, as well as regular breaks for rest, food, or to use the restroom. To reduce eye strain or cognitive overload, it might help to install a blue light filter on your computer screen.

Those with complex chronic illness in college can usually qualify for services designed to grant those with disabilities equal access to education. That can mean extended time for exams, being able to take a test in a quieter environment or a testing center with fewer distractions, or having a notetaker take class notes for you. After an initial letter from a doctor, the university's disability services sends an accommodation letter given to a student's professors each semester, and there's no need to disclose any uncomfortable medical information to the faculty.

In her 1969 book *On Death and Dying*, psychiatrist Elisabeth Kübler-Ross put forth her famous theory of the five stages of grief, which begins with Denial, proceeds toward Anger, Bargaining, and Depression, and ends with the ultimate goal of Acceptance. Just as learning to accept the death of a loved one is a vital part of the grief process, the loss of a version of oneself, whether temporarily or permanently, follows a similar process of grief. That's why it can be useful for those with complex chronic diseases to seek care with a therapist to complement their multidisciplinary medical care with a cardiologist, rheumatologist, or perhaps many others. Adjusting one's expectations can be a path toward finding joy in a new life, which harnesses newfound limitations rather than fighting against them.

In her book *The Phenomenology of Illness*, philosopher Havi Carel examines an idea from the philosopher S. Kay Toombs, explaining that with chronic illness we have five major losses: the loss of wholeness, certainty, control, freedom, and familiarity. These losses, residing inside the concept of *illness*, cannot be contained in the medical or clinical definition of a disease. Disease is the bureaucratic language of lab tests, specialist referrals, insurance reimbursement. What is or is not reported on a medical chart cannot define us. Illness is our own first-person subjective experience, our own life as directly lived.

Carel herself was diagnosed with a Lymphangioleiomyomatosis (LAM), a rare lung disease that leads to respiratory failure. Following the diagnosis, she wrote, "My future has folded in on itself." But it sparked her interest in pursuing the meaning of her new life, and to find a philosophical footing within it. Therefore, if an illness is viewed as an opportunity to philosophize, it "can be seen as dramatically changing the ways of being that are available to a person and thus prompting, provoking, or inviting them to modify their being."

Such an endeavor of reflective coping recalls the ancient Greek notion that philosophy is about learning how to die. Here it is not a physical death of the body itself, but at least a death of some vital part of the living self. Suspending a previous life requires learning how to bear illness well—living alongside a disability, reckoning with the pain, and processing the shock and sadness. She recalls the Stoic thinker Epictetus, who wrote, "What is it to bear a fever well? Not to blame God or man; not to be afflicted at that which happens, to expect death well and nobly, to do what must be done."

And modifying one's own being can mean harnessing the illness as an opportunity for post-traumatic growth, taking the perspective away from long-term goals in the future, and focusing in on the present moment, dwelling in the current experience. We can cope with illness by keeping stock of what is still possible.

In that respect, she finds sustenance in the words of Friedrich Nietzsche, whose own struggle with neurological disease reoriented his philosophical outlook:

"It was as if I discovered life anew, myself included; I tasted all the good things, even the small ones, as no other could easily taste them—I turned my will to health, to life, into my philosophy...the years when my vitality was at its lowest were when I stopped being a pessimist."

FORGING A REALISTIC HOPE

One frame of mind that has guided me through some of my worst relapses has been what business consultant Jim Collins has called the "Stockdale Paradox." It's the idea that in times of greatest hardship, you "must maintain unwavering faith that you can and will prevail in the end, regardless of the difficulties, and at the same time, have the discipline to confront the most brutal facts of your current reality, whatever they might be." Collins coined the term in his 2001 book *Good to Great* after interviewing Admiral James Stockdale, who had been the senior ranking U.S. military officer held at the infamous "Hanoi Hilton" prison in Vietnam. Collins asked Stockdale who among the captives was most likely to die, and the admiral—who became a Stoic philosopher after the war—said, "Oh, that's easy. The optimists." Prisoners who naively clung to a falsely positive belief of being released and home by Christmas were the ones most likely to succumb to hopelessness and despair. When the arbitrary deadline they'd held in their minds came and went, a physical and emotional collapse ensued.

The survivors had a different mindset, one which could combine acknowledgment of their circumstances' stark reality with an unwavering faith that things can and would get better. Holding those two ideas together simultaneously is also a way of navigating the uncertainty and unrelenting hell of a disease you don't deserve.

The concept of "unwavering faith" aligns closely with that of hope. And while religious practices have preached the benefits and rewards of faith and hope for millennia, science and the field of positive psychology are beginning to unravel its utility as well. In his book *The Anatomy of Hope*, Dr. Jeremy Groopman distinguishes between two types of hope: true hope and false hope. Groopman, a physician-scientist at Harvard Medical School, was once a patient navigating the complexities of chronic pain. Initially, as both a patient and a practitioner, Groopman struggled with the idealized versions of hope reflected in pop culture and its ties to uncorroborated follies like wishful thinking. However, after experiencing his own success with hope, Groopman decided to take his subjective experience and explore the idea of hope objectively through science. Groopman's book reflects his decades of research on the effect true hope has on people facing serious and terminal illnesses. According to Groopman, two key elements of hope—belief and expectation—can be cardinal components of the placebo response. When patients hope for or expect a treatment, the placebo effect can trigger a cascade of pain-relieving endorphins in the brain.

In alignment with hope, researchers have been exploring mindset as a way to elicit progress across many disciplines. Originally investigated in the classroom by psychologist Carol Dwerk, a concept known as *growth mindset* explores how believing in one's potential and growth helps us see a future where options exist, allowing us to set expectations and goals. That, in turn, changes our behavior. According to researchers in the field, growth mindset is in juxtaposition to a fixed mindset where goal-oriented effort is blunted by an inescapable view of oneself and the world. Fixed mindset might include giving up easily and having low expectations for oneself. A growth mindset includes developing flexible beliefs about one's potential, seeing challenges as learning experiences and opportunities, and having resilience to setbacks. But could growth mindset be applied to our wellness as well? Could hope change our brains? Could our mindset change our actions? Some wellness programs seem to think so. Other medical practitioners believe positive psychology around health is akin to the placebo effect. And while there is a small, but growing body of research to affirm that mindset can affect physiological outcomes and symptom severity, science has not shown us that mindset can alter serious disease processes such as cancer outcomes. However, if a growth mindset can promote goal-setting and includes being open to trying a new potential treatment, the outcome may change. Mix that with a dose of endorphin release, and you might have the ingredients for progress.

While mindset, hope, and optimism may have their place as supportive therapies for people experiencing chronic conditions, it's also important to acknowledge how harmful these seemingly positive tools can be if used incorrectly or taken to the extreme. When medical practitioners, friends, or family offer these tools in a package that claims to cure disease, they unwittingly minimize the complexity and seriousness of devastating physical disease. When doctors suggest a change in mindset without properly acknowledging or medically addressing the depth of their patient's physical pain and suffering, patients can be left feeling the opposite of hope.

These facts are particularly challenging in the face of contested or invisible diseases such as Long Covid. There may be great potential to keeping hope and seeing your future abilities as flexible. But I've always found these truths must be balanced with pacing, respecting one's boundaries, and an acceptance of reality. A true hope.

And perhaps the truest hope I know is a faith in the resilience of regular people with lived experience of a problem to gather together, of strangers unified through no other connection than their own shared suffering. I believe in the power of connective technologies that provide a forum for shared communities to flourish, propping each other up with mutual support when whole systems seem to have failed. I believe in the power of regular people to help write or reform policy, and to endeavor in a collective effort ceaselessly to try and change the world. And whether we actually change it or not, I believe in that collective striving, in the sparks that fly out from the friction of striking against a rocky adversary. I believe in that tension of idealism and cynicism, which is our constant, universal act of becoming in this world.

Acknowledgments

First and foremost, I'm thankful to the dozens who generously gave their time for long interviews, especially in the midst of a strange disease. I hope this book helps you feel validated in your experience and contributes to a more just world.

I am grateful to my parents, Mary and Tom Prior. None of this is possible without your love, commitment, and unfailing belief. I'm so fortunate to have won the lottery with such deeply supportive and caring parents. They hosted me and cooked for me during several months of this project, enabling me to focus solely on writing. And both reviewed multiple drafts with me line by line along the way, improving anything from minor punctuation errors to major structural changes.

Elizabeth Weaver, my researcher, was like a divine gift. She serves on the neuroscience faculty at Georgia State as an adjunct working on interdisciplinary policy and administration, lives with ME/CFS, and moonlights with her firm, Brain Wheel, providing research and design for non-fiction books. I couldn't have dreamt up a better partner and friend to soldier through brainstorming, early drafts, and the formidable process of endnotes with me. She stepped in to help write a few sections as well, including on shame, infection theory, gaslighting, sexism, and hope. I will cherish our masked-up, socially distanced outdoor selfies as cicadas chirped in the Georgia summer and the air sparked with ideas and fireflies.

I thank my high school teachers Scott Daniel, the man who taught me to love to write, and Pam Stanescu, whose love of learning thrilled all of us and whose love toward me ensured I wouldn't fail in my moments of greatest need.

I am grateful to the institutions which have anchored my life, and built me into the writer, advocate, and man I am today.

At CNN, I was blessed with thousands of colleagues engaged in the collective endeavor to tell the story of our times with rigor, thoughtfulness, and high professionalism. From all of you, I have learned the craft of journalism, singing in many keys across quick news hits, lengthy reported features, and producing for television. You've all pushed me to be both dreamily ambitious and meticulously careful. Colleen Covino and Cristina Hernandez fought to give me the writing opportunities that could fill my soul. A dedicated editor, Brandon Griggs, helped my feature stories shine with cinematic pace and flair. Ben Tinker, David Allan, Katia Hetter, Justin Lear, Saeed Ahmed, Calvin Houts, Linda Rathke, and Damon Peebles all cultivated my creativity and curiosity. Thank you to CNN for giving me several months off to start this manuscript.

The Stanford Medicine X community, founded by the visionary Dr. Larry Chu, inspired me to believe that patient voices matter. The values of the collective ensured I didn't ever feel alone or abnormal in living with a chronic illness. My fellow ePatients affirmed that experiences of suffering can be a profound gift to others, making us *more than* and not *less than*. Medicine X has been a catalyst to write about patients from the spectrum of diseases who were unwilling to accept the status quo and took it upon themselves to innovate, advocate, and instigate a more inclusive healthcare future in which patients take their rightful place at the center. Their examples, including Doug Lindsay, Andrea Downing, Grace Anne Dorney Koppel, and dozens of others, are a light.

ACKNOWLEDGMENTS

The #MEAction Network, founded by Jennifer Brea and Beth Mazur, has provided a global structure pushing for health equity for those with ME. It's one of the great honors of my life to work with so many talented, altruistic people on a mission far larger than myself.

Thank you to my agent Jennifer Weis, for believing in this project with such enthusiasm, and injecting confidence into me from our very first meeting. I thank Pam Weintraub for introducing me to Jennifer after ScienceWriters 2020.

At Post Hill Press, thank you to Debra Englander for spotting the potential for this book when it was in its early proposal stages and offering me the opportunity to publish it. Thank you to managing editor Heather King for ably managing each stage of the process, and to Devan Murphy for her superb and thoughtful copyedits, strengthening the manuscript. And thank you to Devon Brown for being sharp in running publicity.

I felt deeply supported by my fact checker, Maya Dusenbery, herself the author of *Doing Harm*, a book about contested illnesses and sexism in medicine. She brought extraordinary subject matter expertise as we tightened the scientific facts in the text. Any remaining errors are, of course, my own.

My friends Doug Lindsay, David Tuller, Brian Vastag, Beth Mazur, Imraan Sumar, Travis Preston, and Cecily McMillan all walked with me in this journey, joyfully supporting long workshop sessions and pushing to make the book everything it could be. Though she didn't live to see the pandemic or this book, I felt the presence of the late Cindy Shepler, who for years had breathed hope into me and preached the interconnectedness of all autoimmune diseases. At Hutchins State Jail in Texas, James McMillan reviewed and discussed the progress of the book with me weekly.

Chapter 1: A Future in Jeopardy

"It's important to remember,"...Alex Azar, "Remarks by President Trump, Vice President Pence, and Members of the Coronavirus Task Force in Press Conference," transcript of speech delivered at the James S. Brady Press Briefing Room, February 29, 2020, https://trumpwhitehouse.archives.gov/briefings-statements/remarks-president-trump-vice-president-pence-members-coronavirus-task-force-press-conference-2/.

*But like seven million others in the U.S....*Rafael Harpaz, MD, MPH, "Prevalence of Immunosuppression Among US Adults, 2013," JAMA Network, December 20, 2016, https://jamanetwork.com/journals/jama/fullarticle/2572798.

"To keep new cases from entering our shores,"...Donald Trump, "Read President Trump's Speech on Coronavirus Pandemic: Full Transcript," *The New York Times*, March 11, 2020, https://www.nytimes.com/2020/03/11/us/politics/trump-coronavirus-speech.html.

I have told the stories...Ryan Prior, "I Can't Shake Covid-19: Warnings from Young Survivors Still Suffering," CNN, July 19, 2020, https://www.cnn.com/2020/07/18/health/long-term-effects-young-people-covid-wellness/index.html; "Redefining Covid-19: Months after Infection, Patients Report Breathing Difficulty, Excessive Fatigue," CNN, September 13, 2020, https://www.cnn.com/2020/09/13/health/long-haul-covid-fatigue-breathing-wellness/index.html; "Covid-19's Effects Include Seizures and Movement Disorders—Even in Some

Moderate Cases, Study Finds," CNN, December 10, 2020, https://www.cnn.com/2020/12/10/health/effects-on-the-brain-covid-19-wellness/index.html; "A Third of Covid-19 Survivors Suffer 'Brain Disease,' Study Shows," CNN, April 6, 2021, https://www.cnn.com/2021/04/06/health/covid-neurological-psychological-lancet-wellness/index.html.

*A 2009 study of 369 SARS survivors...*Marco Ho-Bun Lam, Yun-Kwok Wing, Mandy Wai-Man Yu, Chi-Ming Leung, Ronald C. W. Ma, Alice P. S. Kong, W.Y. So, Samson Yat-Yuk Fong, and Siu-Ping Lam, "Mental Morbidities and Chronic Fatigue in Severe Acute Respiratory Syndrome Survivors: Long-Term Follow-Up," *Archives of Internal Medicine* 169, no. 22 (2009): 2142-47. doi:10.1001/archinternmed.2009.384.

irreversible paralysis in about 1 in 200 patients..."Poliomyelitis," World Health Organization, July 22, 2019, https://www.who.int/news-room/fact-sheets/detail/poliomyelitis.

the virus also caused post-polio syndrome..."Post-Polio Syndrome," Centers for Disease Control and Prevention, Last modified September 23, 2021, https://www.cdc.gov/polio/what-is-polio/pps.html.

Ebola killed more than a third..."2014-2016 Ebola Outbreak in West Africa," Centers for Disease Control and Prevention, Last modified March 8, 2019, https://www.cdc.gov/vhf/ebola/history/2014-2016-outbreak/index.html.

*more than 70 percent of survivors...*Nell G Bond, Donald S Grant, Sarah T Himmelfarb, Emily J Engel, Foday Al-Hasan, Michael Gbakie, Fatima Kamara, Lansana Kanneh, Ibrahim Mustapha, Adaora Okoli, William Fischer, David Wohl, Robert F Garry, Robert Samuels, Jeffrey G Shaffer, John S Schieffelin, "Post-Ebola Syndrome Presents With Multiple Overlapping Symptom Clusters: Evidence From an Ongoing Cohort Study in Eastern Sierra Leone," Oxford Academic, September 15, 2021, https://academic.oup.com/cid/article/73/6/1046/6209860.

*the CDC released a study of 292 Covid-19 patients...*Mark W. Tenforde, Sara S. Kim, Christopher J. Lindsell, Erica Billig Rose, Nathan I.

Shapiro, D. Clark Files, Kevin W. Gibbs, Heidi L. Erickson, Jay S. Steingrub, Howard A. Smithline, et al., IVY Network Investigators, CDC COVID-19 Response Team, "Symptom Duration and Risk Factors for Delayed Return to Usual Health among Outpatients with Covid-19 in a Multistate Health Care Systems Network—United States, March–June 2020," *Morbidity and Mortality Weekly Report* 69, no. 30 (June 2020): 993-98. https://doi.org/10.15585/mmwr.mm6930e1.

one in ten people were sick for at least three weeks…"How Long Does Covid-19 Last?" ZOE Covid Study, June 6, 2020, https://covid.joinzoe.com/post/covid-long-term…

I wrote a story for USA Today…Ryan Prior, "Viewpoint: The Real Story of Chronic Fatigue Syndrome," *USA Today*, October 02, 2012, https://www.usatoday.com/story/college/2012/10/02/viewpoint-the-real-story-of-chronic-fatigue-syndrome/37397751/.

I wrote about Stanford's Ron Davis…Ryan Prior, "He Pioneered Technology That Fueled the Human Genome Project. Now His Greatest Challenge Is Curing His Own Son," CNN, May 12, 2019, https://www.cnn.com/2019/05/12/health/stanford-geneticist-chronic-fatigue-syndrome-trnd/index.html.

I profiled Doug Lindsay…Ryan Prior, "This College Dropout Was Bedridden for 11 Years. Then He Invented a Surgery and Cured Himself," CNN, July 27, 2019, https://www.cnn.com/2019/07/27/health/doug-lindsay-invented-surgery-trnd/index.html.

a series of features on Dr. David Fajgenbaum…Ryan Prior, "This Med Student Was Given Last Rites Before Finding a Treatment That Saved His Life. His Method Could Help Millions," CNN, September 14, 2019, https://www.cnn.com/2019/09/14/health/castleman-fajgenbaum-chasing-my-cure-wellness-trnd/index.html; "After Saving His Own Life With a Repurposed Drug, a Professor Reviews Every Drug Being Tried Against Covid-19. Here's What He's Found," CNN, July

27, 2020, https://www.cnn.com/2020/06/27/health/coronavirus-treat-ment-fajgenbaum-drug-review-scn-wellness/index.html.

up to 100 million long haulers worldwide...Chen Chen, Spencer R. Haupert, Lauren Zimmermann, Xu Shi, Lars G. Fritsche, and Bhramar Mukherjee, "Global Prevalence of Post-Acute Sequelae of COVID-19 (PASC) or Long COVID: A Meta-Analysis and Systematic Review," *MedRXiv*, November 16, 2021, https://www.medrxiv.org/content/10.1 101/2021.11.15.21266377v1.

More than 150 million Americans...Christine Buttorff, Teague Ruder, and Melissa Bauman, "Multiple Chronic Conditions in the United States," RAND, May 31, 2017, https://www.rand.org/pubs/tools/TL221.html.

Chapter 2: A Surprising Problem

A growing body of research shows that..."Introduction to COVID-19 Racial and Ethnic Health Disparities," Center for Disease Control and Prevention, last modified December 10, 2020, https://www.cdc.gov/coronavirus/2019-ncov/community/health-equity/racial-eth-nic-disparities/index.html; Wyatt Koma, Samantha Artiga, Tricia Neuman, Gary Claxton, Matthew Rae, Jennifer Kates, and Josh Michaud, "Low-Income and Communities of Color at Higher Risk of Serious Illness if Infected with Coronavirus," KFF, May 2020, https://www.kff.org/coronavirus-covid-19/issue-brief/low-income-and-communities-of-color-at-higher-risk-of-serious-illness-if-in-fected-with-coronavirus/; Neal Marquez, MPH1; Julie A. Ward, MN, RN2; Kalind Parish, MA3; et al, "COVID-19 Incidence and Mortality in Federal and State Prisons Compared With the US Population, April 5, 2020, to April 3, 2021," JAMA Network, October 6, 2021, https://jamanetwork.com/journals/jama/fullarticle/2784944; Irene Gibson, Marc R. Rosenblum, Bryan Baker, and Alexander Eastman, "COVID-19 Vulnerability by Immigration Status," US Department of Homeland Security, May 2021, https://www.dhs.gov/sites/default/files/publications/immigration-statistics/research_reports/research_paper_covid-19_vulnerability_by_immigration_status_may_2021.pdf; Lindsey Dawson, Ashley Kirzinger, and Jennifer Kates, "The Impact of the Covid-19 Pandemic on LGBT People," KFF, March, 11, 2021. https://www.kff.org/coronavirus-covid-19/poll-finding/the-impact-of-the-covid-19-pandemic-on-lgbt-people/.

*experts worry they will be further alienated...*Elizabeth Cooney, "Researchers Fear People of Color May Be Disproportionately Affected by Long Covid," STAT, May 10, 2021, https://www.statnews.com/2021/05/10/with-long-covid-history-may-be-repeating-itself-among-people-of-color/.

more severe outcomes occurred in communities of color..."Risk for COVID-19 Infection, Hospitalization, and Death By Race/Ethnicity," Center for Disease Control and Prevention, last modified March 25, 2022, https://www.cdc.gov/coronavirus/2019-ncov/covid-data/investigations-discovery/hospitalization-death-by-race-ethnicity.html.

*Amy Carrillo, a forty-three-year-old from Kansas...*Amy Carrillo, Interview by Ryan Prior, August 23, 2021.

*Michael Sieverts was another...*Michael Sieverts, Interview by Ryan Prior, 2021.

*Clare Daly, thirty-eight, the chief product officer...*Clare Daly, Interview by Ryan Prior, August 23, 2021.

*Yvette Walker, a fifty-one-year-old writer...*Yvette Walker, Interview by Ryan Prior, August 26, 2021.

*Kimberly Shay's taste buds...*Kimberly Shay, Interview by Ryan Prior, August 23, 2021.

*Courtney Garvin, a singer and guitarist...*Courtney Garvin, Interview by Ryan Prior, August 23, 2021.

And for Molly Adams…Molly Adams, Interview by Ryan Prior, August 23, 2021.

Bahtiyar Bozkurt, a thirty-seven-year-old engineer…Bahtiyar Bozkurt, Interview by Ryan Prior, August 24, 2021.

Cali Wilson was similarly…Cali Wilson, Interview by Ryan Prior, August 23, 2021.

Marie, a twenty-six-year-old hacker…Marie, Interview by Ryan Prior, August 26, 2021.

Rabia Jaffer, a teacher from Toronto…Rabia Jaffer, Interview by Ryan Prior, August 23, 2021.

Marjorie Roberts, a life coach from Georgia…Marjorie Roberts, Interview by Ryan Prior, August 23, 2021.

Dani Mortell had summited…Dani Mortel, Interview by Ryan Prior, August 23, 2021.

Kimberley Grant, a social worker…Kimberley Grant, Interview by Ryan Prior, August 23, 2021.

For Alexis Misko, an occupational therapist…Alexis Misko, Interview by Ryan Prior, August 23, 2021.

Esther La Russa, a cashier from Illinois…Esther La Russa, Interview by Ryan Prior, August 23, 2021.

Felipe Andrés Araya Casanova, a thirty-two-year-old…Felipe Andrés Araya Casanova, Interview by Ryan Prior, August 23, 2021.

Eva Amat, a fifty-one-year-old secretary…Eva Amat, Interview by Ryan Prior, August 27, 2021.

Joni Savolainen, a thirty-five-year-old…Joni Savolainen, Interview by Ryan Prior, August 21, 2021.

*Jenna, a young woman working...*Jenna, Interview by Ryan Prior, August 27, 2021.

*Enya Vermeyen, a mathematics teacher...*Enya Vermeyen, Interview by Ryan Prior, August 24, 2021.

*Deborah Lee, a twenty-six-year-old...*Deborah Lee, Interview by Ryan Prior, August 23, 2021.

*James McMillan, incarcerated...*James McMillan, Interview by Ryan Prior, August 26, 2021.

*Amanda Finley experienced...*Amanda Finley, Interview by Ryan Prior, October 21, 2021.

*Álvaro Rial, thirty...*Álvaro Rial, Interview by Ryan Prior, August 24, 2021.

MIS-C had appeared in about 7,880 U.S. pediatric Covid cases..."Health Department-Reported Cases of Multisystem Inflammatory Syndrome in Children (MIS-C) in the United States," Centers for Disease Control and Prevention, Last modified (May 2022), https://covid.cdc.gov/covid-data-tracker/#mis-national-surveillance.

*have less access to post-acute hospital care...*Moses J.E. Flash et al, "Disparities in Post-Intensive Care Syndrome During the Covid-19 Pandemic: Challenges and Solutions." NEJM, 2020, https://doi.org/10.1056/CAT.20.0568.

in an estimated 10 percent to 30 percent of those infected..."Prevalence of Ongoing Symptoms Following Coronavirus (COVID-19) Infection in the UK: 1 April 2021," Office for National Statistics, April, 1, 2021, https://www.ons.gov.uk/peoplepopulationandcommunity/healthandsocialcare/conditionsanddiseases/bulletins/prevalenceofongoingsymptomsfollowingcoronaviruscovid19infectionintheuk/1april2021; Jennifer K. Logue, BS1; Nicholas M. Franko, BS1; Denise J. McCulloch, MD, MPH1; et al, "Sequelae in Adults at 6 Months After COVID-19 Infection," JAMA Network, February 19, 2021, https://

jamanetwork.com/journals/jamanetworkopen/fullarticle/2776560; Chen Chen, Spencer R. Haupert, Lauren Zimmermann, Xu Shi, Lars G. Fritsche, Bhramar Mukherjee, "Global Prevalence of Post-Acute Sequelae of COVID-19 (PASC) or Long COVID: A Meta-Analysis and Systematic Review," PubMed, April 2022, https://pubmed.ncbi.nlm.nih.gov/35429399/.

The Covid death rate in most developed countries..."Mortality Analyses," Johns Hopkins University & Medicine, last modified April 26, 2022, https://coronavirus.jhu.edu/data/mortality.

the World Health Organization's report in February 2020..."Report of the WHO-China Joint Mission on the Coronavirus Disease 2019 (COVID-19)," World Health Organization, February 2020, https://www.who.int/docs/default-source/coronaviruse/who-china-joint-mission-on-covid-19-final-report.pdf.

*One of those citizen scientists was...*Ben Zimmer, "Long hauler: When Covid-19's Symptoms Last and Last," *Wall Street Journal*, January 1, 2021, https://www.wsj.com/articles/long-hauler-when-covid-19s-symptoms-last-and-last-11609524809.

Chapter 3: A Groundswell of Patient Activism

*Fiona Lowenstein, a twenty-six-year-old freelance writer...*Fiona Lowenstein, Interview by Ryan Prior, 2021.

*The op-ed recounted how the coronavirus...*Fiona Lowenstein, "I'm 26. Coronavirus Sent Me to the Hospital." *New York Times,* March 23, 2020, https://www.nytimes.com/2020/03/23/opinion/coronavirus-young-people.html.

*This second piece, published on April 13, 2020...*Fiona Lowenstein, "We Need to Talk About What Coronavirus Recoveries Look Like," *The New York Times,* April 13, 2020, https://www.nytimes.com/2020/04/13/opinion/coronavirus-recovery.html.

Alison Sbrana had fallen ill...Alison Sbrana, Interview by Ryan Prior, 2021.

10 percent with mono develop long-term symptoms...D S Buchwald, et al. "Acute Infectious Mononucleosis: Characteristics of Patients Who Report Failure to Recover," *The American Journal of Medicine* 109,7 (2000): 531-7, doi:10.1016/s0002-9343(00)00560-x https://pubmed. ncbi.nlm.nih.gov/11063953/.

women more than twice as likely as men...Lawrence B. Afrin, Joseph H. Butterfield, Martin Raithel, and Gerhard J. Molderings, "Often Seen, Rarely Recognized: Mast Cell Activation Disease – a Guide to Diagnosis and Therapeutic Options," *Annals of Medicine* 48, no. 3: 190-201. https://doi.org/10.3109/07853890.2016.1161231; I.J. Bakken et al, "Two Age Peaks in the Incidence of Chronic Fatigue Syndrome/ Myalgic Encephalomyelitis: A Population-Based Registry Study from Norway," *BMC Med* 12, 167 (October 2014), https://doi.org/10.1186/ s12916-014-0167-5; B. H. Shaw, L. E. Stiles, K. Bourne, E. A. Green, et al, "The Face of Postural Tachycardia Syndrome – Insights From a Large Cross-Sectional Online Community-Based Survey," *Journal of Internal Medicine* 286, no 4 (October 2019): 438-448. https://doi. org/10.1111/joim.12895.

Hannah Davis, who was a thirty-two-year-old...Hannah Davis, Interview by Ryan Prior, 2021.

Gina Assaf, a design strategist...Gina Assaf, Interview by Ryan Prior, 2021.

Lisa McCorkell, twenty-eight...Lisa McCorkell, Interview by Ryan Prior, 2021.

Hannah Wei, a Canadian product consultant...Hannah Wei, Interview by Ryan Prior, 2021.

Athena Akrami, a neuroscientist...Athena Akrami, Interview by Ryan Prior, 2021.

The survey generated 640 responses...Gina Assaf, Hannah Davis, Lisa McCorkell, Hannah Wei, O'Neil Brooke, Athena Akrami, Ryan Low et al, "What Does Covid-19 Recovery Actually Look Like?" Patient-Led Research Collaborative, May 11, 2020, https://patientresearchcovid19.com/research/report-1/.

a June 4, 2020 piece in The Atlantic...Ed Yong, "Covid-19 Can Last for Several Months," *The Atlantic*, June 4, 2020, https://www.theatlantic.com/health/archive/2020/06/covid-19-coronavirus-longterm-symptoms-months/612679/.

an archeologist named Elisa Perego...Elisa Perego, Email to Ryan Prior, August 16, 2021.

Claire Hastie, a corporate consultant...Claire Hastie, Interview by Ryan Prior, 2021.

Long Covid is just as likely to stem from a mild case...Jennifer Logue et al, "Sequelae in Adults at 6 Months After COVID-19 Infection," *JAMA Network* 4, (February 2021), https://jamanetwork.com/journals/jamanetworkopen/fullarticle/2776560.

"Message in a Bottle" YouTube video...LongCovidSOS Team, "Message in a Bottle Long Covid SOS," United Kingdom, 2020, https://www.youtube.com/watch?v=IIeOoS_A4c8.

published a British Medical Journal *opinion piece*...Amali Lokugamage, Sharon Taylor, and Clare Rayner, "Patients' Experiences of 'Longcovid' Are Missing from the NHS Narrative," B*MJ Opinion*, July 10, 2020. https://blogs.bmj.com/bmj/2020/07/10/patients-experiences-of-long-covid-are-missing-from-the-nhs-narrative/.

a virtual press conference about Covid-19...Adeeba Kamarulzaman, Anthony Fauci, Claudio Fenizia, Andrew Hill, Kristen Marks, and Carina Marquez, "Official Press Conference: COVID-19 Conference Highlights (Thursday, 9 July)," International AIDS Conference,

July 9, 2020, conference recording https://www.youtube.com/watch?v=UMmT48IC0us.

Terri Wilder, a social worker…Terri Wilder, Interview by Ryan Prior, 2021.

organized a virtual meeting…Brianna Sacks, "COVID Is Making Younger, Healthy People Debilitatingly Sick For Months. Now They're Fighting For Recognition," Buzzfeed, Last modified August 25, 2020, https://www.buzzfeednews.com/article/briannasacks/covid-long-haulers-who-coronavirus.

They documented more than 200 symptoms…Hannah E. Davis, Gina S. Assaf, Lisa McCorkell, Hannah Wei, Ryan J. Low, Yochai Re'em, Signe Redfield, Jared P. Austin, and Athena Akrami, "Characterizing Long Covid in an International Cohort: 7 Months of Symptoms and Their Impact," MedRxiv, (2020), 2020.12.24.20248802.

published in the peer reviewed journal…Hannah E. Davis et al, "Characterizing Long COVID in an International Cohort: 7 months of Symptoms and Their Impact," *The Lancet* 38, (August 2021), https://www.thelancet.com/journals/eclinm/article/PIIS2589-5370(21)00299-6/fulltext.

Perego published an article…Felicity Callard and Elisa Perego, "How and Why Patients Made Long Covid," Short Communication, *Social Science & Medicine* 268, (2020), doi:10.1016/j.socscimed.2020.113426

The WHO reported 1.65 million social media mentions…"Update on Clinical Long-Term Effects of Covid-19," World Health Organization, Last Modified March 26, 2021, https://www.who.int/docs/default-source/coronaviruse/risk-comms-updates/update54_clinical_long_term_effects.pdf?sfvrsn=3e63eee5_8.

Chapter 4: Patients Become the Experts

Our word patient *comes to us from the Latin "patiens"*…J Neuberger, "Do We Need a New Word for Patients? Let's Do Away with 'Patients.'" [In eng]. *BMJ (Clinical research ed.)* 318, no. 7200 (1999): 1756-57. https://doi.org/10.1136/bmj.318.7200.1756. https://pubmed.ncbi.nlm.nih.gov/10381717.

Fiona Lowenstein, Body Politic's founder…Fiona Lowenstein, Interview by Ryan Prior, 2021.

series of one-pagers…"Post-COVID Conditions: Information for Healthcare Providers," Centers for Disease Control and Prevention," Last modified July 9, 2021, https://www.cdc.gov/coronavirus/2019-ncov/hcp/clinical-care/post-covid-conditions.html.

NIH Director Francis Collins highlighted…Francis Collins, "Trying to Make Sense of Long Covid Syndrome," NIH ed., (2021), https://directorsblog.nih.gov/2021/01/19/trying-to-make-sense-of-long-covid-syndrome/.

penned a Wall Street Journal *opinion piece*…Jeremy Devine, "The Dubious Origins of Long Covid," *Wall Street Journal*, March 22, 2021. https://www.wsj.com/articles/the-dubious-origins-of-long-covid-11616452583.

"Mickey Mouse science at best"…Mike Mariani, "The Great Gaslighting: How COVID Longhaulers are Still Fighting for Recognition," *The Guardian*, February 3, 2022, https://www.theguardian.com/society/2022/feb/03/long-covid-fight-recognition-gaslighting-pandemic.

"It's possible that I would not be studying…Ziyad Al-Aly, Interview by Ryan Prior, 2021.

His team's study was published…Ziyad Al-Aly, Yan Xie, and Benjamin Bowe, "High-Dimensional Characterization of Post-Acute Sequelae of Covid-19," *Nature* 594, no. 7862 (2021): 259-64, https://doi.org/10.1038/s41586-021-03553-9.

Kramer, an Oscar-nominated screenwriter...Randy Shilts, *And the Band Played On: Politics, People, and the Aids Epidemic.* New York, New York: St Martin's Press, 2007.

the 2012 documentary How to Survive a Plague...David France, "How to Survive a Plague," 2012. https://surviveaplague.com.

*Davis resonated with a different type...*Hannah Davis, Interview Ryan Prior, 2021.

*Claire Hastie, the founder...*Clarie Hastie, Interview by Ryan Prior, 2021.

a global conference on Long Covid..."Long COVID Forum: 9-10 December 2020," International Severe Acute Respiratory and emerging Infection Consortium, last modified December 9, 2020, https://isaric.org/event/long-covid-joint-research-forum-virtual-events-9-10-december-2020/.

*an agenda identifying research priorities...*G. Carson and Long Covid Group, "Research Priorities for Long Covid: Refined Through an International Multi-Stakeholder Forum," *BMC Med* 19, no 84 (2021), https://bmcmedicine.biomedcentral.com/articles/10.1186/s12916-021-01947-0.

*"I have these weird neurological symptoms...*Chelsea Cirruzzo, "'It's Personal and It's Policy': Sen. Tim Kaine Details His Bout with Long Covid," U.S. News & World Report, March 24, 2021. https://www.usnews.com/news/health-news/articles/2021-03-24/tim-kaine-on-bout-with-long-covid-its-personal-and-its-policy.

testify in front of the House Energy and Commerce Committee..."The Long Haul: Forging a Path through the Lingering Effects of COVID-19," The Subcommittee on Health of the Committee on Energy and Commerce, April 28, 2021, recorded hearing, https://energycommerce.house.gov/committee-activity/hearings/hearing-on-the-long-haul-forging-a-path-through-the-lingering-effects-of.

For her testimony, Lisa McCorkell…Lisa McCorkell, Interview by Ryan Prior, 2021.

interim guidelines for treating post-Covid conditions…"Evaluating and Caring for Patients with Post-Covid Conditions: Interim Guidance," Centers for Disease Control and Prevention, Last Modified June 14, 2021, https://www.cdc.gov/coronavirus/2019-ncov/hcp/clinical-care/post-covid-index.html.

And Alison Sbrana, seven years after…Alison Sbrana, Interview by Ryan Prior, 2021.

"It is beautiful to see this…"A Brief but Spectacular Take on Chronic Illness," PBS, https://www.pbs.org/video/brief-but-spectacular-1619123266/.

$1.15 billion check for research…Francis S. Collins, "NIH launches new initiative to study 'Long COVID'," National Institutes of Health, February 23, 2021, https://www.nih.gov/about-nih/who-we-are/nih-director/statements/nih-launches-new-initiative-study-long-covid.

introduce the Covid-19 Long Haulers Act…"Nearly $100m in Long Covid Funding Introduced in Congress," PRNewswire Press Release, May 27, 2021. https://www.prnewswire.com/news-releases/nearly-100m-in-long-covid-funding-introduced-in-congress-301301363.html.

champion was Emily Taylor…Emily Taylor, Interview by Ryan Prior, 2021.

Only about a fifth…"Beyond Myalgic Encephalomyelitis/Chronic Fatigue Syndrome: Redefining an Illness," National Academy of Medicine, 2015, https://nap.nationalacademies.org/catalog/19012/beyond-myalgic-encephalomyelitischronic-fatigue-syndrome-redefining-an-illness.

allocating $15 million annually…"Estimates of Funding for Various Research, Condition, and Disease Categories (RCDC)," National Institute of Health, June 25, 2021, https://report.nih.gov/funding/categorical-spending#/.

the Covid-19 and Pandemic Response Centers of Excellence Act… "As Omicron Cases Are Detected In New York, Gillibrand Pushes For Creation Of Covid-19 And Pandemic Response Centers Of Excellence To Prepare For Future Variants And Help Prevent Public Health Emergencies," Kirsten Gillibrand U.S. Senator for New York, December 5, 2021, https://www.gillibrand.senate.gov/news/press/release/as-omicron-cases-are-detected-in-new-york-gillibrand-pushes-for-creation-of-covid-19-and-pandemic-response-centers-of-excellence-to-prepare-for-future-variants-and-help-prevent-public-health-emergencies.

The White House Covid-19 Health Equity Task Force… "Presidential COVID-19 Health Equity Task Force," U.S. Department of Health and Human Services Office of Minority Health, October 2021, https://www.minorityhealth.hhs.gov/assets/pdf/HETF_Report_508_102821_9am_508Team%20WIP11-compressed.pdf.

recommendations presented by Davis and McCorkell… Hannah Davis and Lisa McCorkell, "White House Covid-19 Equity Task Force Presentation", Patient-Led Research Collaborative, 2021, https://docs.google.com/presentation/d/1QoXnLSwV-tB7Le9R9SiF6Xouf9q0t-TOuQKF3KYZIf1Q/mobilepresent?slide=id.gdd634b6900_0_101.

More than eighty Long Covid clinics… Erika Edwards, "Inside 'Post-Covid' Clinics: How Specialized Centers are Trying to Treat Long-Haulers," *NBC News*, March 1, 2021, https://www.nbcnews.com/health/health-news/inside-post-covid-clinics-how-specialized-centers-are-trying-treat-n1258879.

Dr. David Putrino, the Director of Rehabilitation Innovation… David Putrino, Interview with Ryan Prior, 2022.

Chapter 5: A Lifelong Mission

In a press conference to launch..."CDC Launches 'Get Informed. Get Diagnosed. Get Help.' Campaign," CDC Newsroom Press Release, November 3, 2006, https://www.cdc.gov/media/pressrel/r061103.htm.

*an important study by Dr. Ian Lipkin...*Harvey J. Alter et al, "A Multicenter Blinded Analysis Indicates No Association between Chronic Fatigue Syndrome/Myalgic Encephalomyelitis and either Xenotropic Murine Leukemia Virus-Related Virus or Polytropic Murine Leukemia Virus," *ASM Journals* 3, no 5 (September 2012), https://journals.asm.org/doi/full/10.1128/mBio.00266-12.

a more personal USA Today *column...*Ryan Prior, "Viewpoint: The Real Story of Chronic Fatigue Syndrome," *USA Today*, October 02, 2012, https://www.usatoday.com/story/college/2012/10/02/viewpoint-the-real-story-of-chronic-fatigue-syndrome/37397751/.

The Atlantic *published a story...*Nicole Allan, "Who Will Tomorrow's Historians Consider Today's Greatest Inventors?" *The Atlantic*, November 2013, https://www.theatlantic.com/magazine/archive/2013/11/the-inventors/309534/.

*the most serious journalistic investigation into ME/CFS...*Hillary Johnson, *Osler's Web: Inside the Labyrinth of the Chronic Fatigue Syndrome Epidemic*, (United States: Penguin US, 1996).

*patients had a host of abnormalities...*Klimas NG, Salvato FR, Morgan R, Fletcher MA. "Immunologic Abnormalities in Chronic Fatigue Syndrome," *J Clin Microbiol* 28, (June 1990:1403-10), doi: 10.1128/jcm.28.6.1403-1410.1990. PMID: 2166084; PMCID: PMC267940.

published a paper in the journal Annals of Internal Medicine...D. Buchwald, P. R. Cheney, D. L. Peterson, B. Henry, S. B. Wormsley, A. Geiger, D. V. Ablashi, et al, "A Chronic Illness Characterized by Fatigue, Neurologic and Immunologic Disorders, and Active Human

Herpesvirus Type 6 Infection," [In eng]. *Ann Intern Med* 116, no. 2 (January 1992): 103-13, https://doi.org/10.7326/0003-4819-116-2-103.

*just 43 percent of the $23 million...*June Gibbs Brown, "Audit of Costs Charged to the Chronic Fatigue Syndrome Program at the Centers for Disease Control and Prevention (CIN: A-04-98-04226)," Office of Inspector General, May 10, 1999, https://oig.hhs.gov/oas/reports/region4/49804226.pdf.

*Davis sought two NIH grants...*Olga Khazan, "The Tragic Neglect of Chronic Fatigue Syndrome," *The Atlantic*, October 8, 2015, https://www.theatlantic.com/health/archive/2015/10/chronic-fatigue-patients-push-for-an-elusive-cure/409534/.

*30 percent of medical school curricula...*Mark Peterson, Thomas W. Peterson, Sarah Emerson, Eric Regalbuto, Meredyth Evans, and Leonard Jason, "Coverage of CFS within U.S. Medical Schools," *Universal Journal of Public Health* 1, no. 4 (2013). https://doi.org/10.13189/ujph.2013.010404.

*Discover magazine called Lipkin...*Grant Delin, "Discover Interview: The World's Most Celebrated Virus Hunter, Ian Lipkin," *Discover Magazine*, 2012, https://www.discovermagazine.com/health/discover-interview-the-worlds-most-celebrated-virus-hunter-ian-lipkin.

*a $766,000 grant to complement...*Olga Khazan, "The Tragic Neglect of Chronic Fatigue Syndrome."

her own documentary about the disease...Unrest, Directed by Jennifer Bea, Shella Films, 2017.

*Newt Gingrich had penned a 2015 op-ed...*Newt Gingrich, "Newt Gingrich: Double the N.I.H. Budget," *The New York Times*, April 22, 2015, https://www.nytimes.com/2015/04/22/opinion/double-the-nih-budget.html.

an estimated $17 to $24 billion…Leonard A. Jason, Mary C. Benton, Lisa Valentine, Abra Johnson, and Susan Torres-Harding, "The Economic Impact of ME/CFS: Individual and Societal Costs," [In eng], *Dynamic medicine*, 7 (2008): 6-6. https://doi.org/10.1186/1476-5918-7-6.

a similar disease, multiple sclerosis, had only about one-third…Ashley R. Valdez, Elizabeth E. Hancock, Seyi Adebayo, David J. Kiernicki, Daniel Proskauer, John R. Attewell, Lucinda Bateman, et al, "Estimating Prevalence, Demographics, and Costs of ME/CFS Using Large Scale Medical Claims Data and Machine Learning," [In English]. *Frontiers in Pediatrics* 6, (2019), https://doi.org/10.3389/fped.2018.00412.

ought to have been $203 million annually…Arthur Mirin, Mary Dimmock, and Leonard Jason, "Research Update: The Relation between ME/CFS Disease Burden and Research Funding in the USA," Work 66, no. 2 (2019): 277–82. https://doi.org/10.3233/WOR-203173.

slot at the Stanford Medicine X conference…Ryan Prior, "Epatient Ignite! Ryan Prior," In Stanford Medicine X, 8:56, 2017. https://www.youtube.com/watch?v=wajdSXwRaJA.

in Man's Search for Meaning…Viktor Frankl, *Man's Search for Meaning* (Boston: Beacon Press, 1959).

Rilke's semi-autobiographical novel…Rainer Maria Rilke, "For the Sake of a Single Poem," *In the Notebooks of Malte Laurids Brigge* (Austria-Hungary, 1910).

six times greater risk of suicide…Dr. Emmert Roberts et al, "Mortality of people with chronic fatigue syndrome: a retrospective cohort study in England and Wales from the South London and Maudsley NHS Foundation Trust Biomedical Research Centre (SLaM BRC) Clinical Record Interactive Search (CRIS) Register," *The Lancet* 387, no 10028 (April 2016): 1638-1643, https://www.thelancet.com/journals/lancet/article/PIIS0140-6736(15)01223-4/fulltext.

Buddhist nun Pema Chödrön…Pema Chödrön, *When Things Fall Apart: Heart Advice for Difficult Times* (Boston: Shambhala: 2000).

Chapter 6: We Predicted This

Leonard Jason, a professor of psychology...Leonard Jason, Interview with Ryan Prior, 2021.

a four-year study of mononucleosis...Leonard A Jason, Joseph Cotler, Mohammed F Islam, Madison Sunnquist, and Ben Z Katz, "Risks for Developing Myalgic Encephalomyelitis/Chronic Fatigue Syndrome in College Students Following Infectious Mononucleosis: A Prospective Cohort Study," *Clinical Infectious Diseases*, (2020), https://doi.org/10.1093/cid/ciaa1886.

"If you look at all the pandemics...Leonard Jason, Interview by Ryan Prior, 2021.

a century of post-infectious syndromes...Mohammed Islam, Joseph Cotler, and Leonard Jason, "Post-Viral Fatigue and Covid-19: Lessons from Past Epidemics," Review. *Fatigue: Biomedicine, Health & Behavior* 8, no. 20 (2020): 61-69, https://www.tandfonline.com/doi/epub/10.1080/21641846.2020.1778227.

a 2006 study conducted in Australia...I. Hickie, T. Davenport, D. Wakefield, U. Vollmer-Conna, B. Cameron, S. D. Vernon, W. C. Reeves, and A. Lloyd, "Post-Infective and Chronic Fatigue Syndromes Precipitated by Viral and Non-Viral Pathogens: Prospective Cohort Study," [In eng]. *BMJ* 333, no. 7568 (Sep 16, 2006): 575, https://doi.org/10.1136/bmj.38933.585764.AE.

A study in Houston, Texas...Kristy O. Murray et al, "Survival Analysis, Long-Term Outcomes, and Percentage of Recovery Up to 8 Years Post-Infection Among the Houston West Nile Virus Cohort," *PloS One* 9, no 7 (July 2014), https://www.ncbi.nlm.nih.gov/pmc/articles/PMC4108377/.

28 percent of those recovering from Ebola...Himiede W Wilson et al, "Post-Ebola Syndrome Among Ebola Virus Disease Survivors in Montserrado County, Liberia 2016," *BioMed Research International*, (June 2018), https://www.ncbi.nlm.nih.gov/pmc/articles/PMC6046154/.

It showed that 40 percent of patients reported chronic fatigue...Marco Ho-Bun Lam, Yun-Kwok Wing, Mandy Wai-Man Yu, Chi-Ming Leung, Ronald C. W. Ma, Alice P. S. Kong, W.Y. So, Samson Yat-Yuk Fong, and Siu-Ping Lam, "Mental Morbidities and Chronic Fatigue in Severe Acute Respiratory Syndrome Survivors: Long-Term Follow-Up," *Archives of Internal Medicine* 169, no. 22 (2009): 2142-47, doi:10.1001/archinternmed.2009.384.

there's likely some kind of a wrench in the machinery...Gerwyn Morris and Michae Maes, "Mitochondrial Dysfunctions in Myalgic Encephalomyelitis / Chronic Fatigue Syndrome Explained by Activated Immuno-Inflammatory, Oxidative and Nitrosative Stress Pathways," *Metab Brain Dis* 29, (March 2014): 19-36, https://link.springer.com/article/10.1007/s11011-013-9435-x.

Dr. David Putrino was in a unique position...David Putrino, Interview by Ryan Prior, 2022.

redesign the Precision Recovery app...L. Tabacof, C. Kellner, E. Breyman, S. Dewil, S. Braren, L. Nasr, J. Tosto, M. Cortes, and D. Putrino, "Remote Patient Monitoring for Home Management of Coronavirus Disease 2019 in New York: A Cross-Sectional Observational Study," [In eng]. *Telemed J E Health* 27, no. 6 (Jun 2021): 641-48, https://doi.org/10.1089/tmj.2020.0339.

people with Long Covid have hypocapnia...Jamie Wood et al, "Levels of end-tidal carbon dioxide are low despite normal respiratory rate in individuals with long COVID," *Journal of Breath Research* 16, no 1 (December 2021), https://iopscience.iop.org/article/10.1088/1752-7163/ac3c18/pdf.

Chapter 7: Covid for Christmas

my most personal story for CNN...Ryan Prior, "My Friend Chose an Assisted Death in Switzerland. Her Dying Wish was to Tell You Why,"

CNN, June 7, 2020, https://www.cnn.com/2020/06/07/health/cindy-shepler-assisted-death-wellness-trnd/index.html.

a book by Franciscan priest Richard Rohr...Richard Rohr, *The Universal Christ* (New York: Convergent Books, 2019).

Social Security Disability Insurance and Supplemental Security Income... "Chart Book: Social Security Disability Insurance," Center on Budget and Policy Priorities, Last Modified February 12, 2021, https://www.cbpp.org/research/social-security/social-security-disability-insurance-0.

40 percent of workers...Martin J. Walsh and William W. Beach, "National Compensation Survey: Employee Benefits in the United States," U.S. Bureau of Labor Statistics, March 2021, https://www.bls.gov/ncs/ebs/benefits/2021/employee-benefits-in-the-united-states-march-2021.pdf.

words of the Greek playwright Aeschylus...Edith Hamilton, *The Greek Way* (New York: W.W. Norton & Company, 2010), https://books.google.com/books/about/The_Greek_Way.html?id=D3QwvF3GWOkC.

In his classic book Man's Search for Meaning...Viktor Frankl, *Man's Search for Meaning* (Boston: Beacon Press, 1959).

Susan Sontag's famous collection of essays...Susan Sontag, *Illness as Metaphor* (New York: Knopf Doubleday Publishing Group, 1978).

Chapter 8: Unraveling the Mystery

Athena Akrami was unique...Athena Akrami, Interview by Ryan Prior, 2021.

a preprint paper offering a set of hypotheses...Russell N. Low et al, "A Cytokine-based Model for the Pathophysiology of Long COVID Symptoms," *OSF Preprints*, (November 2020), https://doi.org/10.31219/osf.io/7gcnv.

*Dr. Noah Greenspan, a pulmonary rehab therapist…*Noah Greenspan, Interview by Ryan Prior, 2021.

produce a documentary film…Long Haul, directed by Noah Greenspan (A Pulmonary Wellness Foundation Film, 2021), 38:36, https://www. longhaul.movie/.

*Michael VanElzakker is a neuroscientist…*Michael VanElzakker, Interview by Ryan Prior & Elizabeth Weaver, 2021.

*he published his vagus nerve infection hypothesis…*Michael B.VanElzakker, "Chronic Fatigue Syndrome from Vagus Nerve Infection: A Psychoneuroimmunological Hypothesis," *Medical Hypothesis* 81, no 3 (September 2013): 414-423, https://www.science-direct.com/science/article/abs/pii/S0306987713002752?via%3Dihub.

*he and microbiologist Amy Proal authored…*Amy D. Proal and Michael B. VanElzakker, "Long Covid or Post-Acute Sequelae of Covid-19 (PascPASC): An Overview of Biological Factors That May Contribute to Persistent Symptoms," [In English], *Frontiers in Microbiology* 12, (June 2021), https://doi.org/10.3389/fmicb.2021.698169.

*intrigued by one German study…*Jakob Matschke, Marc Lütgehetmann, Christian Hagel, Jan P. Sperhake, Ann Sophie Schröder, Carolin Edler, Herbert Mushumba et al, "Neuropathology of Patients with Covid-19 in Germany: A Post-Mortem Case Series," *The Lancet Neurology* 19, no. 11 (2020): 919-29, https://doi.org/10.1016/S1474-4422(20)30308-2.

*Geralyn Lucas, an author…*Geralyn Lucas, Interview by Ryan Prior, 2021.

*long haulers reported feeling partially or totally recovered…*Ryan Prior, "Some Covid-19 Long Haulers Say Vaccines May Be Relieving Their Symptoms. Researchers Are Looking into It," CNN, March 4, 2021, https://www.cnn.com/2021/04/03/health/long-haulers-vaccine-wellness/index.html.

Several informal patient surveys…"The Impact of COVID Vaccination on Symptoms of Long Covid. An international survey of 900 people with Lived Experience," LongCovidSOS, Last accessed April 9, 2022, https://3ca26cd7-266e-4609-b25f-6f3d1497c4cf.filesusr.com/ugd/8bd4fe_a338597f76bf4279a851a7a4cb0e0a74.pdf; RUN-DMC / Gez Medinger, "First Vaccine Reaction Data For Long Covid | Pfizer, AstraZeneca and Moderna Analyzed," YouTube, February 23, 2021, https://www.youtube.com/watch?v=Lio2ByLW4WE; Francis Stead Sellers, "Could Long Covid Unlock Clues to Chronic Fatigue and Other Poorly Understood Conditions?" *Washington Post*, November 7, 2021, https://www.washingtonpost.com/health/2021/11/07/long-covid-fatigue-research/.

16.6 percent of long haulers…Viet-Thi Tran, Elodie Perrodeau, Julia Saldanha, Isabelle Pane, and Philippe Ravaud, "Efficacy of Covid-19 Vaccination on the Symptoms of Patients with Long Covid: A Target Trial Emulation Using Data from the Compare E-Cohort in France," *The Lancet*, Preprint, (September 2021), https://papers.ssrn.com/sol3/papers.cfm?abstract_id=3932953.

Akiko Iwasaki, a professor…Akiko Iwasaki, Interview by Ryan Prior, 2021.

the most notable patient survey…"The Impact of COVID Vaccination on Symptoms of Long Covid. An International Survey of 900 People with Lived Experience," LongCovidSOS, Last Accessed April 9, 2022, https://3ca26cd7-266e-4609-b25f-6f3d1497c4cf.filesusr.com/ugd/8bd4fe_a338597f76bf4279a851a7a4cb0e0a74.pdf.

recruited participants into the study…Caroline Leiber, "In Search of Answers About Long Covid-19, Scientists Turn to Social Media," *Yale School of Medicine*, January 26, 2022. https://medicine.yale.edu/news-article/in-search-of-answers-about-long-covid-19-scientists-turn-to-social-media/.

Chapter 9: The NIH Goes Big

Dr. Avindra Nath, the clinical director…Avindra Nath, Interview by Ryan Prior, 2021.

About 10 percent of its funding…"Budget," National Institute of Health. Last modified June 29, 2020, https://www.nih.gov/about-nih/what-we-do/budget.

supporting basic research…"Basic Research—Digital Media Kit," National Institutes of Health, last modified March 12, 2021, https://www.nih.gov/news-events/basic-research-digital-media-kit.

led to the gene editing tool CRISPR…Loureiro, Alexandre, and Gabriela Jorge da Silva, "CRISPR-Cas: Converting A Bacterial Defence Mechanism into A State-of-the-Art Genetic Manipulation Tool," *Antibiotics* 8, no.1 (January 2019):18, https://doi.org/10.3390/antibiotics8010018.

Nath began giving presentations…Anonymous source at the NIH. Personal communication to Ryan Prior, October 13, 2020.

Researching Covid to Enhance Recovery, or RECOVER Initiative…"Recover: Researching Covid to Enhance Recovery," Recover, Last accessed April 26, 2022, https://recovercovid.org.

problems that had plagued early research…Ryan Prior, "Here's How to Design Drug Trials to Defeat the Next Pandemic," CNN, July 4, 2021, https://www.cnn.com/2021/07/04/health/drug-trials-covid-pandemic/index.html.

Some 92 percent of the trials…Kushal T. Kadakia et al, "Leveraging Open Science to Accelerate Research," *The New England Journal of Medicine*, (April 2021), https://www.nejm.org/doi/full/10.1056/NEJMp2034518.

a large UK trial showing…Dylan Scott, "How the UK Found the First Effective Covid-19 Treatment — and Saved a Million Lives," *Vox*,

April 26, 2021, https://www.vox.com/22397833/dexamethasone-coronavirus-uk-recovery-trial.

NIH director Francis Collins said..."The Long Haul: Forging a Path through the Lingering Effects of Covid-19," United States Congress House Energy and Commerce Committee, April, 2021.

*said Dr. Walter Koroshetz...*Walter Koroshetz, Interview by Ryan Prior & Elizabeth Weaver, 2021.

*Karyn Bishof, the founder...*Karyn Bishof, Interview by Ryan Prior, October 26, 2021.

*Harvard's Michael VanElzakker...*Michael VanElzakker, Interview by Ryan Prior & Elizabeth Weaver, 2021.

*Mt. Sinai's David Putrino...*David Putrino, Interview by Ryan Prior, 2022.

*a study on high-intensity interval training...*TK https://anesthesiology.duke.edu/?p=857965

a panel discussion on Long Covid..."Understanding Long COVID: The Unseen Public Health Crisis," Harvard T.H. Chan School of Public Health, educational video, November 19, 2021, https://www.hsph.harvard.edu/event/understanding-long-covid-the-unseen-public-health-crisis/.

*the PLRC published an open letter...*The Patient-Led Research Collaborative, "Open Letter Regarding the RECOVER Initiative to Study Long COVID," Patient-Led Research Collaborative, November 29, 2021, https://patientresearchcovid19.com/open-letter-regarding-the-recover-initiative-to-study-long-covid/.

*the Body Politic had urged the NIH...*Fiona Lowenstien and Angela Vázquez, "Open Letter to the NIH," Body Politic, April 22, 2021, https://www.wearebodypolitic.com/bodytype/2021/4/22/open-letter-to-nih.

half of long haulers met the diagnostic criteria…C Kedor et al, "Chronic COVID-19 Syndrome and Chronic Fatigue Syndrome (ME/CFS) Following the First Pandemic Wave in Germany—A First Analysis of a Prospective Observational Study," MedRXiv, (February 2021), https://www.medrxiv.org/content/10.1101/2021.02.06.21249256v1.

Chapter 10: Gaslighting, Disbelief, and the Search for Answers

Oxford University Press named it…"Word of the Year 2018: Shortlist," Oxford Languages, 2018, https://languages.oup.com/word-of-the-year/2018-shortlist/.

women's unexplained physical symptoms are often "all in their heads"… Diane E. Hoffmann and Anita J. Tarzian, "The Girl Who Cried Pain: A Bias against Women in the Treatment of Pain," *SSRN*, (2001), https://doi.org/http://dx.doi.org/10.2139/ssrn.383803.

as journalist Maya Dusenbery…Maya Dusenbery, *Doing Harm: The Truth About How Bad Medicine and Lazy Science Leave Women Dismissed, Misdiagnosed and Sick* (San Francisco, California: HarperOne, 2018).

83 percent of women with chronic pain…"Women in Pain Survey," The National Pain Report and For Grace, September 12, 2014, https://www.surveymonkey.com/results/SM-P5J5P29L/.

wait longer for pain treatment…Esther H Chen et al, "Gender Disparity in Analgesic Treatment of Emergency Department Patients with Acute Abdominal Pain," *Academic Emergency Medicine: Official Journal of the Society for Academic Emergency Medicine* 15, no 5 (2008): 414-8, https://pubmed.ncbi.nlm.nih.gov/18439195/.

women have historically been underrepresented…Carolyn M Mazure and Daniel P Jones, "Twenty Years and Still Counting: Including Women as Participants and Studying Sex and Gender in Biomedical

Research," *BMC Women's Health* 15, no 94 (October 2015), https://pubmed.ncbi.nlm.nih.gov/26503700/.

for those with poorly understood conditions...Anne Werner and Kirsti Malterud, "It is Hard Work Behaving as a Credible Patient: Encounters Between Women with Chronic Pain and Their Doctors," *Social Science & Medicine* 57, no 8 (2003): 1409-1419, https://pubmed.ncbi.nlm.nih.gov/12927471/.

Researchers from the University of Virginia showed...Kelly M. Hoffman, Sophie Trawalter, Jordan R. Axt, and M. Norman Oliver, "Racial Bias in Pain Assessment and Treatment Recommendations, and False Beliefs About Biological Differences between Blacks and Whites," *Proceedings of the National Academy of Sciences of the United States of America* 113, no. 16 (2016): 4296-301. https://www.pnas.org/doi/full/10.1073/pnas.1516047113.

A 2013 review published in the American Medical Association's Journal of Ethics...Ronald Wyatt, "Pain and Ethnicity," *Virtual Mentor* 15, no 5 (May 2013): 449-454, https://journalofethics.ama-assn.org/article/pain-and-ethnicity/2013-05.

In her paper "The Sociology of Gaslighting"...Paige L. Sweet, "The Sociology of Gaslighting," *American Sociological Review* 84, no. 5 (2019): 851-75, https://doi.org/10.1177/0003122419874843.

The UK-based Long Covid Support organization ran a survey..."Long Covid Assessment Services Patient Feedback," Long Covid, May 2021, https://drive.google.com/file/d/1UFEUgw1LEOz4Jx_wGwknrtbGH t0TkZk9/view.

Guardian *columnist George Monbiot found*...George Monbiot, "We're About to See a Wave of Long Covid. When Will Ministers Take It Seriously?" *The Guardian*, January 21, 2021, https://www.theguardian.com/commentisfree/2021/jan/21/were-about-to-see-a-wave-of-long-covid-when-will-ministers-take-it-seriously.

presentation that an Oxford psychiatrist gave...Michael Sharpe, "Post COVID-19 Syndrome (long Covid),"Swiss Re, February 2021, https://www.swissre.com/dam/jcr:788aa287-7026-430a-8c14-f656421b6e71/swiss-re-institute-event-secondary-covid19-impacts-presentation-michael-sharpe.pdf.

wrote a follow-up column...George Monbiot, "Apparently Just by Talking About It, I'm Super-Spreading Long Covid," *The Guardian*, April 14, 2021, https://www.theguardian.com/commentisfree/2021/apr/14/super-spreading-long-covid-professor-press-coverage.

Showing that this occurs...Staci Stevens et al, "Cardiopulmonary Exercise Test Methodology for Assessing Exertion Intolerance in Myalgic Encephalomyelitis/Chronic Fatigue Syndrome," *Frontiers in Pediatrics* 6, (September 2018), https://www.ncbi.nlm.nih.gov/pmc/articles/PMC6131594/

publication of the PACE Trial...P. D. White, K. A. Goldsmith, A. L. Johnson, L. Potts, R. Walwyn, J. C. DeCesare, H. L. Baber, et al, "Comparison of Adaptive Pacing Therapy, Cognitive Behaviour Therapy, Graded Exercise Therapy, and Specialist Medical Care for Chronic Fatigue Syndrome (Pace): A Randomised Trial," *The Lancet* 377, no. 9768 (2011): 823-36, https://doi.org/10.1016/S0140-6736(11)60096-2.

The study became mired in controversy...Julie Rehmeyer, "Bad Science Misled Millions with Chronic Fatigue Syndrome. Here's How We Fought Back," *STAT*, September 21, 2016, https://www.statnews.com/2016/09/21/chronic-fatigue-syndrome-pace-trial/.

A report by the UK-based ME Association..."ME/CFS Illness Management Survey Results 'No Decisions About Me without Me,'" ME Association, May 2015, https://meassociation.org.uk/wp-content/uploads/2015-ME-Association-Illness-Management-Report-No-decisions-about-me-without-me-30.05.15.pdf.

a 15,000-word analysis disputing the study's methods...David Tuller, "Trial by Error: The Troubling Case of the Pace Chronic Fatigue Syndrome Study," Vincent Racaniello ed. *Virology Blog: About Viruses and Viral Disease*, October 21, 2015, https://www.virology.ws/2015/10/21/trial-by-error-i/.

"When I wrote it, I made sure to say...David Tuller, Interview by Ryan Prior, 2021.

sign an open letter to The Lancet...Ronald W. Davis et al, "An Open Letter to The Lancet, again," Virology, February 10, 2016, https://www.virology.ws/2016/02/10/open-letter-lancet-again/.

Patients and independent scientists who analyzed the data...Carolyn E. Wilshire, Kindlon, et al., "Rethinking the Treatment of Chronic Fatigue Syndrome—A Reanalysis and Evaluation of Findings from a Recent Major Trial of Graded Exercise and CBT," *BMC Psychol* 6, no 6 (March 2018), https://bmcpsychology.biomedcentral.com/articles/10.1186/s40359-018-0218-3.

A 2015 report by the U.S. Institute of Medicine..."Beyond Myalgic Encephalomyelitis/Chronic Fatigue Syndrome: Redefining an Illness," National Academy of Medicine, (2015), https://nap.nationalacademies.org/catalog/19012/beyond-myalgic-encephalomyelitischronic-fatigue-syndrome-redefining-an-illness.

the CDC dropped its recommendation...David Tuller, "Trial by Error: The CDC Drops CBT/GET," Vincent Racaniello ed. *Virology Blog: About Viruses and Viral Disease*, July 10, 2017, https://www.virology.ws/2017/07/10/trial-by-error-the-cdc-drops-cbtget/.

The U.S. federal Agency for Healthcare Research and Quality said...Beth Smith et al, "Diagnosis and Treatment of Myalgic Encephalomyelitis/Chronic Fatigue Syndrome," Rockville (MD): Agency for Healthcare Research and Quality, no 219 ((July 2016), https://www.ncbi.nlm.nih.gov/books/NBK379582/.

A similar evidence review…"NICE ME/CFS Guideline Outlines Steps for Better Diagnosis and Management," National Institute for Health and Care Excellence, October 28, 2021, https://www.nice.org.uk/news/article/nice-me-cfs-guideline-outlines-steps-for-better-diagnosis-and-management.

*"I don't know if I can concretely say…*David Lee, Interview by Ryan Prior, 2021.

A 2019 article in the journal BMC Medical Education…David R. Chen and Kelsey C. Priest, "Pimping: A Tradition of Gendered Disempowerment," *BMC Medical Education* 19, no. 345 (October 2019), https://doi.org/10.1186/s12909-019-1761-1.

*instills a fear of making a mistake…*Abraar Karan, "Medical Students Need to be Quizzed, but 'Pimping' Isn't Effective," Statnews, February 3, 2017, https://www.statnews.com/2017/02/03/medical-students-pimping-testing-knowledge/.

*Cynthia Adinig, a thirty-four-year-old graphic designer…*Cynthia Adinig, Interview by Ryan Prior, 2021.

*Albert Camus wrote in 1942…*Albert Camus, *The Myth of Sisyphus* (France: Editions Gallimard, 1942).

Chapter 11: Chronicles of Uncertain Recoveries

*Maneesh Juneja is a consultant…*Maneesh Juneja, Interview by Ryan Prior, 2021.

One doctor wrote him…"Long Covid: How Becoming a Patient Shaped My Thinking as a Futurist," Academy Health, 2021. https://academyhealth.org/professional-resources/training/prof-dev/long-covid-how-becoming-patient-shaped-my-thinking-futurist.

CDC released their guidelines for post-Covid conditions…"Evaluating and Caring for Patients with Post-COVID Conditions: Interim

Guidance," Centers for Disease Control and Prevention, June 14, 2021, https://www.cdc.gov/coronavirus/2019-ncov/hcp/clinical-care/post-covid-index.html

Gay's journey began in March 2020…Mara Gay, Interview by Ryan Prior, 2021.

Desmond Tutu's The Book of Forgiving…D. Tutu and M. Tutu, *The Book of Forgiving: The Fourfold Path for Healing Ourselves and Our World*, (New York: HarperCollins, 2014), https://books.google.com/books?id=RfhNAgAAQBAJ.

Chapter 12: Precursors: ME/CFS and Lyme

Dr. Nancy Klimas treated many…Nancy Klimas, Interview by Ryan Prior, 2022.

It made her recall…Dr. Nancy Klimas, "Long Covid & Post-Viral ME/CFS: Modeling Complex Illnesses," Webinar from Long Covid Alliance, 2021. https://longcovidalliance.org/body-politic-x-dr-nancy-klimas-long-covid-post-viral-me-cfs-modeling-complex-illnesses/.

may miss more than half of cases…Raphael B. Stricker and Lorraine Johnson, "Lyme Disease: Call for a 'Manhattan Project' to Combat the Epidemic," *PLOS Pathogens* 10, no. 1 (2014), https://doi.org/10.1371/journal.ppat.1003796.

the agency estimates…"How Many People Get Lyme Disease?" Centers for Disease Control and Prevention, Last modified January 13, 2021, https://www.cdc.gov/lyme/stats/humancases.html.

10 to 20 percent of those infected remaining ill…John Aucott et al, "Risk of post-treatment Lyme disease in patients with ideally-treated early Lyme disease: A prospective cohort study," *International Journal of Infectious Disease* 116, (March 2022): 230-237, https://www.sciencedirect.com/science/article/pii/S1201971222000352.

Lyme has been the subject of decades of heated debate...Pamela Weintraub, *Cure Unknown: Inside the Lyme Epidemic*, (New York: St. Martin's Press, 2009).

said Dr. John Aucott...John Aucott, Interview by Ryan Prior, 2021.

The team had found elevated levels...John Aucott et al, "CCL19 as a Chemokine Risk Factor for Posttreatment Lyme Disease Syndrome: a Prospective Clinical Cohort Study," *Clinical and Vaccine Immunology* 23, no 9 (September 2016):757-766, https://www.ncbi.nlm.nih.gov/pmc/articles/PMC5014924/.

They also found that gene regulation patterns...Daniel J.B. Clarke et al, "Predicting Lyme Disease From Patients' Peripheral Blood Mononuclear Cells Profiled With RNA-Sequencing," *Frontiers in Immunology* 12, (March 2021), https://www.frontiersin.org/articles/10.3389/fimmu.2021.636289/full.

other Lyme studies of the metabolome...Bryna L Fitzgerald et al, "Metabolic Response in Patients With Post-treatment Lyme Disease Symptoms/Syndrome," *Clinical Infectious Diseases: an official publication of the Infectious Diseases Society of America* 73, no 7 (2021): 2342-2349, https://pubmed.ncbi.nlm.nih.gov/32975577/.

Early autopsy studies by the NIH...Myoung-Hwa Lee et al, "Microvascular Injury in the Brains of Patients with Covid-19," *The New England Journal of Medicine* 384, no 5 (2021): 481-483, https://www.ncbi.nlm.nih.gov/pmc/articles/PMC7787217/.

a German study of patients...Jakob Matschke et al, "Neuropathology of Patients with COVID-19 in Germany: A Post-Mortem Case Series," *The Lancet* 19, no 11 (November 2020): 919-929, https://www.thelancet.com/journals/laneur/article/PIIS1474-4422(20)30308-2/fulltext.

a more robust autopsy study...Daniel Chertow et al, "SARS-CoV-2 infection and persistence throughout the human body and brain,"

Biological Sciences, (December 2021), https://www.researchsquare. com/article/rs-1139035/v1.

*In a 2018 neuroimaging study...*Jennifer M. Coughlin, Ting Yang, Alison W. Rebman, Kathleen T. Bechtold, Yong Du, William B. Mathews, Wojciech G. Lesniak, et al, "Imaging Glial Activation in Patients with Post-Treatment Lyme Disease Symptoms: A Pilot Study Using [11c]Dpa-713 Pet," *Journal of Neuroinflammation* 15, no. 1 (2018): 346, https://doi.org/10.1186/s12974-018-1381-4.

launched a two-year "Crash Course" study..."Crash Course," Stanford Medicine, Last accessed May 2, 2022, https://snyderlabs.stanford.edu/crashcourse/.

Chapter 13: Theory of Everything

*said Dr. Lucinda Bateman...*Lucinda Bateman, Interview by Ryan Prior, 2021.

*Ron Davis, professor of genetics...*Ron Davis, Interview by Ryan Prior & Elizabeth Weaver, 2022.

It published the 2015 report..."Beyond Myalgic Encephalomyelitis/ Chronic Fatigue Syndrome: Redefining an Illness." National Academy of Medicine. https://nap.nationalacademies.org/catalog/19012/beyond-myalgic-encephalomyelitischronic-fatigue-syndrome-redefining-an-illness

*The OMF funded a study of severe ME/CFS...*Chia-Jung Chang et al, "A Comprehensive Examination of Severely Ill ME/CFS Patients," *Healthcare* 9, no. 10 (September 2021): 1290, https://www.mdpi. com/2227-9032/9/10/1290?fbclid=IwAR3OVmfTMmj3RvNdN-ZL3-juIRbPHClmWvUqfi5y8VO7Beass6wWcKoM1lhk.

*they published initial findings...*R. Esfandyarpour, A. Kashi, M. Nemat-Gorgani, J. Wilhelmy, and R. W. Davis, "A Nanoelectronics-

Blood-Based Diagnostic Biomarker for Myalgic Encephalomyelitis/ Chronic Fatigue Syndrome (ME/CFS)," *Proceedings of the National Academy of Sciences* 116, no. 21 (2019): 10250, https://doi.org/10.1073/ pnas.1901274116.

They enrolled Covid-19 patients in a new study...Ronald Tompkins, "Long Covid to ME/CFS A Potential Second Pandemic," Open Medicine Foundation, March 11, 2021, https://www.omf.ngo/ post-covid-syndrome-to-me-cfs/.

She highlighted their ongoing lines of research...Hannah Davis, Hannah Davis. "Long COVID: Current Research & Research Needs," Power-Point Presentation to NIH Recover Initiative, June 2021, https://docs. google.com/presentation/d/1_meYPsbEGS0QHa17Lk2-023zaPxqih-qMMAkP6-QY_RE/edit#slide=id.gd7355e9495_0_173.

complicated two-step...Tracie White, *The Puzzle Solver* (New York: Hachette, 2021).

a new compound called BC 007...Bettina Hohberger et al, "Case Report: Neutralization of Autoantibodies Targeting G-Protein-Coupled Receptors Improves Capillary Impairment and Fatigue Symptoms After COVID-19 Infection," *Front. Med.* 8, (November 2021), https:// www.frontiersin.org/articles/10.3389/fmed.2021.754667/full.

Proal worked with her colleague...Amy Proal, Interview by Ryan Prior & Elizabeth Weaver, 2022.

a preprint in December 2021...Daniel Chertow et al, "SARS-CoV-2 Infection and Persistence Throughout the Human Body and Brain," Research Square, December 20, 2021, https://www.researchsquare. com/article/rs-1139035/v1.

during a Senate health committee hearing...U.S. Senate Committee on Health, Education, Labor & Pensions, Hearing, "Addressing New Variants: A Federal Perspective on the COVID-19 Response," recorded at G50 Dirksen Senate Office Building, January 11, 2022, https://www.

help.senate.gov/hearings/addressing-new-variants-a-federal-perspective-on-the-covid-19-response.

two-thirds showed Epstein-Barr virus reactivation...Jeffrey E. Gold, Ramazan A. Okyay, Warren E. Licht, and David J. Hurley, "Investigation of Long COVID Prevalence and Its Relationship to Epstein-Barr Virus Reactivation," *Pathogens* 10, no. 6 (June 2021): 763, https://www.mdpi.com/2076-0817/10/6/763.

The clots could be a major contributor...Modjtaba Emadi-Baygi et al, "Corona Virus Disease 2019 (COVID-19) as a System-Level Infectious Disease with Distinct Sex Disparities," Frontiers in Immunology12, 778913 (November 2021), https://www.ncbi.nlm.nih.gov/pmc/articles/PMC8667725/.

Dr. David Systrom used a process...Inderjit Singh, MD et al, "Persistent Exertional Intolerance After COVID-19 Insights From Invasive Cardiopulmonary Exercise Testing," *Chest Infections: Original Research* 161, no 1 (January 2022): 54-63, https://www.ncbi.nlm.nih.gov/pmc/articles/PMC8354807

implicated in a number of post-pathogen disease states...D. J. Harrington, "Bacterial Collagenases and Collagen-Degrading Enzymes and Their Potential Role in Human Disease," *Infection and immunity* 64, no. 6 (1996): 1885-1891, https://doi.org/10.1128/iai.64.6.1885-1891.1996. https://pubmed.ncbi.nlm.nih.gov/8675283.

a plethora of structural instabilities...Fraser Henderson, Claudio Austin, Edward Benzel, Paolo Bolognese, Richard Ellenbogen, Clair Francomano, Candace Ireton et al, "Neurological and Spinal Manifestations of the Ehlers–Danlos Syndromes," *American Journal of Medical Genetics*, (2017), https://onlinelibrary.wiley.com/doi/epdf/10.1002/ajmg.c.31549; Fraser Henderson, "Cranio-Cervical Instability in Patients with Hypermobility Connective Disorders." *Journal of Spine* 5, no 2 (2016), DOI:10.4172/2165-7939.1000299.

Proal ran through a few different scenarios..."The Global Interdependence Center – Solve Long Covid Initiative Program Series: Medical Research," Global Interdependence Center, January 7, 2022, https://www.interdependence.org/resources/the-global-interdependence-center-solve-long-covid-initiative-program-series-medical-research/#.YmscnvXMKL8.

a paper in Immunologic Research...Amy D Proal et al, "Immunostimulation in the Treatment for Chronic Fatigue Syndrome/Myalgic Encephalomyelitis," *Immunologic Research* 56, no 2 (2013): 398-412, https://pubmed.ncbi.nlm.nih.gov/23576059/.

*Pretorius and her team found the microclots...*E. Pretorius, M. Vlok, C. Venter et al, "Persistent Clotting Protein Pathology in Long COVID/Post-Acute Sequelae of COVID-19 (PASC) is Accompanied By Increased Levels of Antiplasmin," *Cardiovasc Diabetol* 20, no 172 (2021), https://cardiab.biomedcentral.com/articles/10.1186/s12933-021-01359-7.

*The South African researchers found a strong signal...*Etheresia Pretorius et al, "Combined Triple Treatment of Fibrin Amyloid Microclots and Platelet Pathology in Individuals with Long COVID/Post-Acute Sequelae of COVID-19 (PASC) Can Resolve Their Persistent Symptoms," PREPRINT (Version 1) available at Research Square, (December 2021), https://www.researchsquare.com/article/rs-1205453/v1.

scientist Leslie Norins offered $1 million..."$1 Million Prize for Alzheimer's Disease Germ Announced by Dr. Leslie Norins on Alzgerm.Org," *PRNewswire* Press Release, January 16, 2018. https://www.prnewswire.com/news-releases/1-million-prize-for-alzheimers-disease-germ-announced-by-dr-leslie-norins-on-alzgermorg-300582042.html.

*Epstein-Barr virus was a precursor for multiple sclerosis...*Kjetil Bjornevik, Marianna Cortese, Brian C. Healy, Jens Kuhle, Michael J.

Mina, Yumei Leng, Stephen J. Elledge, et al, "Longitudinal Analysis Reveals High Prevalence of Epstein-Barr Virus Associated with Multiple Sclerosis," *Science* 375, no. 6578 (2022): 296-301, https://doi.org/doi:10.1126/science.abj8222.

One group of experiments led by Ruth Itzhaki...G A Jamieson et al, "Latent Herpes Simplex Virus Type 1 in Normal and Alzheimer's Disease Brains," *Journal of Medical Virology* 33, no 4 (1991): 224-247, https://pubmed.ncbi.nlm.nih.gov/1649907/; Professor Ruth F Itzhaki PhD et al, "Herpes Simplex Virus Type 1 in Brain and Risk of Alzheimer's Disease," *The Lancet* 349, no 9047 (January 1997): 241-244, https://www.sciencedirect.com/science/article/abs/pii/S014067369 6101495.

this finding has been replicated...Matthew A. Wozniak and Ruth F. Itzhaki, "Antiviral Agents in Alzheimer's Disease: Hope for the Future?" *Therapeutic Advances in Neurological Disorders* 3, no. 3 (2010): 141-52, https://doi.org/10.1177/1756285610370069, https://pubmed.ncbi.nlm.nih.gov/21179606.

Although no single lab won..."Nobody finds the Alzheimer's Germ in $1 Million Challenge, but eight researchers split $200K, says Dr. Leslie Norins of Alzheimer's Germ Quest," *PRNewswire*, February 23, 2021, https://www.prnewswire.com/news-releases/nobody-finds-the-alzheimers-germ-in-1-million-challenge-but-eight-researchers-split-200k-says-dr-leslie-norins-of-alzheimers-germ-quest-3012 32177.html.

a large study in 2018 showed that treatment...Nian-Sheng Tzeng, Chi-Hsiang Chung, Fu-Huang Lin, Chien-Ping Chiang, Chin-Bin Yeh, San-Yuan Huang, Ru-Band Lu, et al, "Anti-Herpetic Medications and Reduced Risk of Dementia in Patients with Herpes Simplex Virus Infections—a Nationwide, Population-Based Cohort Study in Taiwan," *Neurotherapeutics* 15, no. 2 (2018): 417-29, https://doi.org/10.1007/s13311-018-0611-x.

a herpes zoster infection...Vincent Chin-Hung Chen, MD, PhD, "Herpes Zoster and Dementia: A Nationwide Population-Based Cohort Study," *Journal of Clinical Psychiatry* 79, no 1 (2018): 16, https://www.psychiatrist.com/jcp/neurologic/dementia/herpes-zoster-and-dementia/.

bacterium associated with gum disease...Stephen S. Dominy, Casey Lynch, Florian Ermini, Malgorzata Benedyk, Agata Marczyk, Andrei Konradi, Mai Nguyen, et al, "*Porphyromonas Gingivalis* in Alzheimer's Disease Brains: Evidence for Disease Causation and Treatment with Small-Molecule Inhibitors," *Science Advances* 5, no. 1 (2019), https://doi.org/doi:10.1126/sciadv.aau3333.

the Alzheimer's Association and representatives..."International Brain Study: Sars-Cov-2 Impact on Behavior and Cognition," Alzheimer's Association Press Release, Last accessed April 7, 2022. https://www.alz.org/research/for_researchers/partnerships/sars-cov2-global-brain-study.

show markedly slowed metabolism...Robert K. Naviaux et al, "Metabolic features of chronic fatigue syndrome," *Biological Sciences* 113, no 37 (August 2016): 5472-5480, https://www.pnas.org/doi/abs/10.1073/pnas.1607571113.

Chapter 14: A New Epidemic of Disability

an annual $17 to 24 billion impact...Jason, "The Economic Impact of ME/CFS: Individual and Societal Costs," *Dynamic Medicine*, https://doi.org/10.1186/1476-5918-7-6.

co-wrote a New York Times *opinion piece*...Fiona Lowenstein and Hannah Davis, "Long Covid Is Not Rare. It's a Health Crisis," *The New York Times*, March 17, 2021, https://www.nytimes.com/2021/03/17/opinion/long-covid.html.

polio was disabling about 35,000 people..."Polio Elimination in the United States," Centers for Disease Control and Prevention, Last mod-

ified September 28, 2021, https://www.cdc.gov/polio/what-is-polio/
polio-us.html.

according to a study by the nation's Office of National Statistics…
"Prevalence of Ongoing Symptoms Following Coronavirus (COVID-
19) Infection in the UK: 1 April 2021," https://www.ons.gov.uk/
peoplepopulationandcommunity/healthandsocialcare/condition-
sanddiseases/bulletins/prevalenceofongoingsymptomsfollowingcoro-
naviruscovid19infectionintheuk/1april2021

*Davis and McCorkell presented the PLRC findings…*Davis, "White
House Covid-19 Equity Task Force Presentation," https://docs.google.
com/presentation/d/1QoXnLSwV-tB7Le9R9SiF6Xouf9q0tTOuQK-
F3KYZIf1Q/mobilepresent?slide=id.gdd634b6900_0_101.

*President Joe Biden said in a Rose Garden speech…*President Biden,
"Remarks by President Biden Celebrating the 31st Anniversary of
the Americans with Disabilities Act," transcript of speech delivered at the Rose Garden, July 26, 2021, https://www.whitehouse.
gov/briefing-room/speeches-remarks/2021/07/26/remarks-by-pres-
ident-biden-celebrating-the-31st-anniversary-of-the-ameri-
cans-with-disabilities-act/.

*a statement from Body Politic praising the move…*Fiona Lowenstein,
"Body Politic and PLRC Statement on Federal Long Covid Disability
Rights Guidance," We Are Body Politic, July 27, 2021, https://www.
wearebodypolitic.com/bodytype/2021/7/27/body-politic-and-pa-
tient-led-research-collaborative-applaud-federal-long-covid-dis-
ability-rights-guidance-on-anniversary-of-americans-with-disabi-
lities-act.

*the codes can get a bit absurd…*Katie Bo Williams, "The 16 Most
Absurd Icd-10 Codes," Healthcare Dive, August 15, 2015, https://www.
healthcaredive.com/news/the-16-most-absurd-icd-10-codes/285737/.

the ICD-10 code U09.9 went live…"New ICD-10-CM code for Post-
COVID Conditions, following the 2019 Novel Coronavirus (COVID-

19)," Centers for Disease Control and Prevention, October 1, 2021, https://www.cdc.gov/nchs/data/icd/announcement-new-icd-code-for-post-covid-condition-april-2022-final.pdf.

the World Health Organization published its case definition…"A Clinical Case Definition of Post COVID-19 Condition by a Delphi Consensus, 6 October 2021," World Health Organization, October 6, 2021, https://www.who.int/publications/i/item/WHO-2019-nCoV-Post_COVID-19_condition-Clinical_case_definition-2021.1

Karyn Bishof, a co-founder of the Long Covid Alliance…Bishof, Karyn. Interview by Ryan Prior, 2021.

"Originally, before Covid…Jayani Delgado, Interview by Ryan Prior, 2021.

just 34 percent of applicants ultimately win benefits…"Chart Book: Social Security Disability Insurance," Center on Budget and Policy Priorities, Last Modified February 12, 2021, https://www.cbpp.org/research/social-security/social-security-disability-insurance-0.

according to a 2014 analysis…David A. Weaver, "Social Security Disability Benefits: Characteristics of the Approved and Denied Populations," *Sage Journals* 32, no 1 (June 2020): 51-62, https://journals.sagepub.com/doi/abs/10.1177/1044207320933538.

according to Rebecca Vallas…Rebecca Vallas, Interview by Ryan Prior, 2021.

the SSA's 1,200 field offices were closed…Jonathan Stein and David A. Weaver, "Half a Million Poor and Disabled Americans Left Behind by Social Security," The Hill, November 15, 2021, https://thehill.com/opinion/finance/581522-half-a-million-poor-and-disabled-americans-left-behind-by-social-security/?rl=1.

1.6 million jobs in the U.S.…Katie Bach, "Is 'Long Covid' Worsening the Labor Shortage?" *Brookings*, January 11, 2022. https://www.brookings.edu/research/is-long-covid-worsening-the-labor-shortage/.

Chapter 15: The ePatient Revolution and Crowdsourcing Research

*Susannah Fox was one of the people…*Susannah Fox, Interview by Ryan Prior, 2021.

*she wrote in a blog post…*Susannah Fox, "Crazy. Crazy. Long Covid. Obvious," Susannah Fox (blog), January 25, 2021, https://susannahfox.com/2021/01/25/crazy-crazy-longcovid-obvious/.

*digital health version of the Cajun Navy…*Susannah Fox "We Need a Digital Health Cajun Navy," Susannah Fox (blog), June 10, 2019, https://susannahfox.com/2019/06/10/we-need-a-digital-health-cajun-navy/.

the launch of the site PatientsLikeMe…"Patients Like Me," Patients Like Me, Last Accessed April 7, 2022. https://www.patientslikeme.com/about.

*self-reported data from 348 users on the site…*Paul Wicks, Timothy E. Vaughan, Michael P. Massagli, and James Heywood, "Accelerated Clinical Discovery Using Self-Reported Patient Data Collected Online and a Patient-Matching Algorithm," *Nature Biotechnology* 29, no. 5 (May 2011): 411-414, https://doi.org/10.1038/nbt.1837.

*a story deBronkart tells in his 2011 TEDx talk…*Dave deBronkart, "Meet E-Patient Dave," TED Talk, 2011, https://www.ted.com/talks/dave_debronkart_meet_e_patient_dave?language=en#t-616926.

*DeBronkart's story ended up on the front page…*Lisa Wangness, "Electronic Health Records Raise Doubt," *The Boston Globe*, April 13, 2009, https://archive.boston.com/news/nation/washington/articles/2009/04/13/electronic_health_records_raise_doubt/.

*"Gimme my damn data…*Dave deBronkart, "A Movement Is Born: 'Gimme My Damn Data,'" Tincture, June 6, 2019, https://tincture.io/a-movement-is-born-gimme-my-damn-data-a8eee0f520c0.

a concept from Wired *magazine co-founder...*Kevin Kelly, "The Natural History of a New Idea." The Technium, Last accessed May 1, 2022, https://kk.org/thetechnium/natural-history/.

*"Crazy. Crazy. Long Covid. Obvious."...*Fox, "Crazy. Crazy. Long Covid. Obvious."

Distilled into ten design principles..."Our Stanford Medicine X Design Principles," Everyone Included, Last accessed May 1, 2022, https://everyoneincluded.org/#design.

*The process begins by empathizing...*Ramunus Balcaitis, "Design Thinking Models. Stanford d.School," *EMPATHIZE@IT EMPATHIZE. DESIGN. BUILD.* June, 2019. https://empathizeit.com/design-thinking-models-stanford-d-school/.

has now raised..."The Power of 10" Drive-in Gala Celebrates Historic Milestone For Emily's Entourage," Emily's Entourage, December 23, 2021, https://www.emilysentourage.org/the-power-of-10-drive-in-ga-la-celebrates-historic-milestone-for-emilys-entourage/?fb-clid=IwAR2jsD7DM5evYY5jqZ1pJAknC6OZqPcKDTPltRvyn-4BVfQ7zIvWlmFuyFQc.

received a quarter-million dollar grant..."The Promise of Patient-Led Research Integration into Clinical Registries and Research," Patient Centered Outcomes Research Institute, Last accessed April 7, 2022, https://www.pcori.org/research-results/2021/promise-patient-led-re-search-integration-clinical-registries-and-research.

They won a $3 million grant..."Patient-Led Research Collaborative Receives $3M in Funding for Long COVID Research from Balvi, a New Fund for High-Impact COVID Projects from Ethereum Co-Found Vitalik Buterin," Patient-Led Research Collaborative, April 22, 2022, https://patientresearchcovid19.com/press-releases/.

Chapter 16: Expectant Hope

in late December 2021...Austin Landis and Reuben Jones, "Long Covid Still a Risk with Omicrons Despite Milder Illness," NY1, December 29, 2021, https://www.ny1.com/nyc/all-boroughs/news/2021/12/29/fauci-interview-long-covid-still-a-risk-with-milder-omicron-cases.

Long Covid is more likely in individuals...C. Cervia et al, "Immunoglobulin Signature Predicts Risk of Post-Acute COVID-19 Syndrome," *Nature Communications* 13, 446 (January 2022), https://www.nature.com/articles/s41467-021-27797-1; Yapeng Su et al, "Multiple Early Factors Anticipate Post-Acute COVID-19 Sequelae," *Cell* 185, no 5 (March 2022): 881-895, https://www.sciencedirect.com/science/article/pii/S0092867422000721.

the chemokine CCL11 being strongly associated...Anthony Fernández-Castañeda et al, "Mild Respiratory SARS-CoV-2 Infection Can Cause Multi-Lineage Cellular Dysregulation and Myelin Loss in the Brain," *BioRxiv* 20, (January 2022), Preprint, https://www.ncbi.nlm.nih.gov/pmc/articles/PMC8764721/.

Karyn Bishof assembled a list...Karyn Bishof n.d., "A Comprehensive Guide for Covid-19 Longhaulers and Physicians: The PASC Master Document," Last accessed April 8, 2022, https://docs.google.com/document/d/1VfENjAiOBKryT-dIOFyU8CyEAAKVR5xk-9WyvlZF-u4M/edit.

Long hauler Sandhya Kamphampati advised...Sandhya Kamphampati, "Being a Covid Long Hauler Taught Me to be Fearless, Push Back, and Take Lots of Notes," *LA Times*, August 5, 202, https://www.latimes.com/science/story/2021-08-05/heres-how-to-effectively-communicate-with-healthcare-professionals.

the Job Accommodation Network...Job Accommodation Network, Last accessed April 7, 2022, https://askjan.org.

famous theory of the five stages of grief...Elisabeth Kübler-Ross, *On Death and Dying* (New York: Macmillan, 1969).

In her book The Phenomenology of Illness...Carel Havi, *Phenomenology of Illness*, 1st ed. (Oxford: OUP Oxford, 2016).

Jim Collins has called the "Stockdale Paradox."...Jim Collins, *Good to Great*, (New York: Harper Business, 2001).

Dr. Jeremy Groopman distinguishes between...Jeremy E. Groopman, *The Anatomy of Hope: How People Prevail in the Face of Illness.* (New York: Random House, 2005).

a concept known as growth mindset...Carol S. Dwerk, *Mindset: The New Psychology of Success*, (New York: Ballantine Books, 2007).

a small, but growing body of research...Alia J Crum et al, "Mind Over Milkshakes: Mindsets, Not Just Nutrients, Determine Ghrelin Response," *Health Psychology: Official Journal of the Division of Health Psychology, American Psychological Association* 30, no 4 (2011): 424-9, https://pubmed.ncbi.nlm.nih.gov/21574706/; Abiola Keller et al, "Does the Perception that Stress Affects Health Matter? The Association with Health and Mortality," *Health Psychology: Official Journal of the Division of Health Psychology, American Psychological Association* 31, no 5 (2012): 677-84, https://pubmed.ncbi.nlm.nih.gov/22201278/; Alia J Crum and Ellen J Langer, "Mind-Set Matters: Exercise and the Placebo Effect," *Psychological Science* 18, no 2 (2007): 165-171, https://dash.harvard.edu/bitstream/handle/1/3196007/Langer_ExcersisePlaceboEffect.pdf?sequence=1%3FviewType=Print&viewClass=Print

science has not shown us that mindset...J. C. Coyne, M. Stefanek, and S. C. Palmer, "Psychotherapy and Survival in Cancer: The Conflict Between Hope and Evidence," *Psychological Bulletin* 133, no 3 (2007): 367–394, https://doi.apa.org/doiLanding?doi=10.1037%2F0033-2909.133.3.367.